# THE 30-DAY CARNIVORE BOOT CAMP

**Quarto.com**

© 2025 Quarto Publishing Group USA Inc.
Text © 2025 Lady Carnivory, LLC

First Published in 2025 by Fair Winds Press,
an imprint of The Quarto Group,
100 Cummings Center, Suite 265-D,
Beverly, MA 01915, USA.
T (978) 282-9590    F (978) 283-2742

29 28 27 26 25    1 2 3 4 5

ISBN: 978-0-7603-9135-8
Digital edition published in 2025
eISBN: 978-0-7603-9136-5

Library of Congress Cataloging-in-Publication Data available.

Design and layout: Laura Shaw Design
Cover Image: Stocksy
Page Layout: Laura Shaw Design
Illustration: Shutterstock

Printed in China

# THE 30-DAY CARNIVORE BOOT CAMP

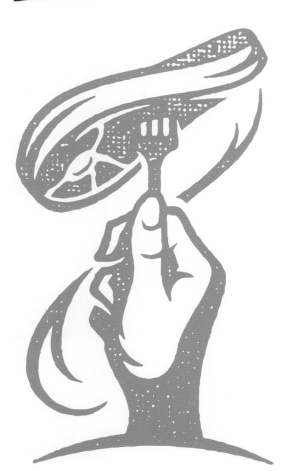

A Beginner's Guide
to Successfully Doing
an All-Meat Lifestyle

—

## JACIE GREGORY

# CONTENTS

# INTRODUCTION

**Thirty days could change your life.
It changed mine.**

**Before I went carnivore,** I would not have described myself as an unhealthy person. Despite the chronic joint pain, debilitating obsessive-compulsive disorder (OCD), and excess of body fat, I really thought my health was just fine.

Like most of us, I grew up eating a standard American diet full of grains, vegetables, and seed oils. As a teenager, I explored a plant-based diet for three years (and coincidentally developed eating disorders). As a young adult, I became enamored with fitness influencers and followed the "If It Fits Your Macros" trend that became popular at that time. If It Fits Your Macros is a nutritional philosophy that believes the type and quality of food that you eat is less important than the ratio of macronutrients (carbs, fat, and protein) that you consume. After that, I tried a more whole foods–based, calories in, calories out approach to eating. Throughout each one of my diet transitions, I never found the energy and ease each new way of eating promised I would achieve.

In 2017, I tried a ketogenic diet for the first time. I stumbled upon this way of eating after a coworker mentioned they were going to try this new high-fat diet. I jumped onto PubMed to look for articles that would prove eating that much fat would kill them and was shocked to find article after article stating the anti-inflammatory benefits of a ketogenic diet. I ate a keto diet for the better part of a year and had amazing weight loss benefits before falling off the wagon.

For the next three years, I struggled to stay on a keto diet, always getting off track if my carb macros wandered outside the tightly controlled rails. It was easy to say to myself, "I'm already one gram over the carb macros, so I might as well eat a dozen donuts."

At the end of 2019, I watched a Joe Rogan podcast that featured Dr. Shawn Baker, an ex-military orthopedic surgeon, sharing the success that he'd found both for himself and his patients through eating a carnivore diet. My takeaway from that interview was that carnivore was an easier version of keto: all of the protein and fat but none of the tracking that worked against me.

At the start of 2020, I decided to do a 30-day carnivore challenge, expecting it to "jump-start" my reentry into a ketogenic way of eating. I was not expecting that going carnivore would completely change my life!

The chronic joint pain I had experienced since I was a teen was gone. The debilitating OCD that made me isolate at home, that I'd tried to treat with prescriptions and therapy for over a decade, was eliminated. Body fat vanished and I finally started to build muscle mass.

Over time, my interest in helping other people discover how to successfully transition to a carnivore diet grew, leading to my carnivore coaching certification in 2021 and nutrition coaching certification in 2022. Over the past couple of years, I have coached hundreds of people through transitioning and sticking to a carnivore way of eating.

Now, four years into eating a mainly carnivore diet, I still enjoy this way of eating. I love having a new understanding of how healthy I can be when I eat the meat I like and can afford and that makes me feel my best. I love the ease and simplicity of shopping for, storing, and cooking a limited variety of foods. I love having consistent energy.

But my carnivore journey has not been linear; a year and a half in I had a catastrophic health decline after being exposed to mold and other biotoxins, which left me walking with a cane and blind in my right eye. Luckily, I found out about chronic inflammatory response syndrome (CIRS), the root cause of the autoimmune issues I was experiencing. CIRS happens when someone is genetically predisposed to not being able to effectively eliminate a biotoxin. When they encounter that biotoxin, it triggers an inflammatory cascade that can lead to further complications. In my case, this was ankylosing spondylitis, a type of autoimmune arthritis that leads to the eventual fusion of your hips to your spine. I spent the next two years recovering from CIRS and the autoimmune disorder it caused.

I am grateful that I remained a carnivore throughout my health setbacks. I know that it helped me have a more accurate view of my healing. Carnivore is an incredibly healing tool because it provides nutritional density while eliminating other possible sources of inflammation. Without the confounding factor of plant toxins and inflammatory seed oils, I was able to understand what my true symptoms were. This book will show you how the quality of your nutrition impacts your health baseline and how healthy you can be in the absence of these extraneous inflammatory factors.

Carnivore gave me other gifts, too. I have made amazing friendships and connections. I met my best friend and my partner through my platform. I have helped family members through their own health problems by encouraging them to eat less seed oils, less grains, less sugar, more meat, and more animal fats. And once I achieved the health and energy I always wanted, I was able to participate in a fitness competition. This was a goal that I harbored in my heart since 2013 but that I never thought I would be able to pursue.

Even more than physical feats, following a carnivore diet allowed me to have better health. I was also able to be more present in my own life and achieve my goals because the time, money, and energy I used to spend managing my health could be used for greater things. Instead of going to doctor appointments, I could go to the gym with my newfound metabolic resilience from eliminating inflammatory toxins from my diet. Instead of feeling lethargic and bingeing Netflix, I could work on creative projects with my improved energy from eating a nutritionally dense diet.

Eating this way allowed me to become the person I always knew I could be. I went from being a person who didn't acknowledge the health problems I experienced on a standard American diet to feeling better than I ever had before. This transformation confirmed my belief in carnivore eating. It also validated my new understanding of what health should really feel like. I am grateful for the balanced view of carnivores I hold today.

After seeing the transformation of so many clients as well, I can recognize its power as an elimination protocol and nutritional reset by removing extraneous toxins and inflammatory agents from the diet. It's not a panacea. It's a possible solution. Once your health baseline—what

your health could be without confounding dietary inflamogens—is revealed, more work may be needed to achieve root-cause healing and long-term wellness.

Between coaching people through carnivore and my new pursuit of sharing awareness about mold illness and chronic inflammatory response syndrome, I have seen people achieve incredible healing. More than anything, I have learned that the pursuit of health is one of the noblest paths we can take in our lives. When we feel our best, we are able to give the best of ourselves to others. We deserve to feel good. And the people we love deserve the best, most present versions of us.

Whether you are looking to adopt this lifestyle to completely transform your health or as an effective yearly reset to reestablish your optimal health baseline, this book will provide you with all the information, resources, and support you need to successfully adopt a carnivore diet for 30 days. I encourage you to read this book with an open mind. While a carnivore diet may not be a long-term lifestyle choice for you, learning how to use it as a nutritional tool to reset your health for 30 days just may change your life too.

**JACIE GREGORY**

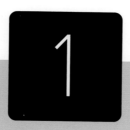

# WHY CARNIVORE?

Despite the confidence with which any expert will tell you they "know" about diet, the complexity of human biology within a rapidly changing modern environment makes research conclusions almost useless. As much as today's media relies on studies to support their claims about nutrition and diet, for every study you can find supporting one dietary choice, you can find another refuting it.

**So why carnivore?** If we cannot prove it is the ideal way of eating, why follow this diet? Why, even, read this book?

Well, if studies convince you, review the Harvard Carnivore Study,[1] with self-reported results from participants who followed a carnivore diet. Look at individual studies showing the benefits of a bioavailable,[2] nutritionally dense diet.[3] Examine the research of Weston A. Price, a dentition inspired to discover why modern teeth seem to decay easily when our ancestors' teeth did not.[4]

Bottom line, there is undeniable evidence for this way of eating. There are indications through the archaeological and anthropological record that our ancestors ate a meat-based diet, such as the Sioux tribes of South Dakota,[5] who ate a diet rich in buffalo meat, the Chukotka of Russia[6], and the Inuit of North America, who survived on the caribou, marine animals, and fish available to them in the Arctic Circle.[7] There are indications, especially through modern anecdotal evidence from both internet forums and the Harvard Carnivore Study[8], that a carnivore diet can improve health.

Besides the ancestral evidence that supports eating more meat, there are nutritional benefits, mental health benefits, and physical health benefits, which we will explore in this chapter. Once you discover and define your reasons for embarking on a new way of eating, it will help you stay on track.

It's well established that our ancestors were hunter-gatherer cultures. Before the rise of agriculture, tribal societies like the Sioux and Chukotka, much like modern-day tribes like the Maasai and Inuit, would have gone out into the wilderness to hunt down meat as their main source of energy. The Maasai can still be visited and studied today in Kenya. The Weston A. Price Foundation still provides up-to-date studies on anthropological evidence[9] of ancestral diets through the dental record. And there is an undoubted correlation between the rise of modern civilization and the rise of chronic diseases.[10]

Cooked meat is likely the reason we evolved to this point,[11] and it points to an interesting question. Is it possible that we can stop the current regression of our evolution by reinstating some of our ancestral eating practices?

# NUTRITION

The primary reasons for starting and sticking to a carnivore diet are because it offers nutritional benefits and makes you feel good. An animal-based diet is rich in protein and fat, which are essential macronutrients necessary for energy and repair. A carnivore diet allows for ketogenic macros—high fat, moderate protein, low carbohydrate—that promote energy production through the metabolism of fat.

Meat is also extremely nutritionally dense; it is packed with all the essential vitamins and minerals you need, like vitamin A, vitamin $B_{12}$, magnesium, and much, much more. Even better, those vitamins are the most bioavailable, which means the body can easily process and use them.

## Understanding Micronutrients and Macronutrients

Nutrients, both micro and macro, play essential roles in many bodily functions. Consuming a nutrient-dense diet can help ensure your body has all the tools and building blocks it needs to perform optimally. A carnivore diet contains all the nutrients that are necessary for optimal brain function, neurotransmitter synthesis, and mood regulation.

**Micronutrients:** These are the nutrients that the body requires in smaller amounts but are vital for numerous physiological processes. Micronutrients include vitamins and minerals. Vitamins are essential for various biochemical reactions in the body, including energy metabolism, immune function, and tissue repair. Minerals are essential for maintaining fluid balance, nerve function, muscle contraction, and bone health.

**Macronutrients:** These are nutrients that the body requires in large amounts. They provide energy via calories to fuel various bodily functions. The three macronutrients are carbohydrates, proteins, and fats. Carbohydrates can be used for energy but can spike blood sugar, leading to inflammation. Proteins are essential for building and repairing tissues as well as providing glucose to the brain in low-carbohydrate environments. Fats provide energy, maintain cell structure, and facilitate absorption of fat-soluble vitamins.

Of the three macronutrients, only carbohydrates are unnecessary for proper nutrition. Your body does need a small amount of glucose, an energy source typically converted from carbohydrates. However, your body can create glucose from protein through a process known as gluconeogenesis. Gluconeogenesis is a metabolic process that synthesizes glucose from amino acids. This process occurs in the liver when glucose availability is low, like when you are fasting or eating a low-carbohydrate diet.

In addition to being a glucose source as needed, protein provides the essential amino acids necessary for many bodily functions. Protein synthesis, enzyme production, hormone regulation, neurotransmitter production, immune function, transport and storage of nutrients, and pH balance all require sufficient protein intake. Your body cannot operate optimally without complete protein consumption.

Unlike plant sources of protein, animal sources of protein are complete, meaning they contain all the essential amino acids. Of the twenty amino acids that make up protein structures, only nine are essential, or absolutely necessary for appropriate bodily functions, because they cannot be synthesized in the body. In plant-based diets, careful combining of different plant protein sources is required to obtain all the amino acids needed.

Most animal-based protein sources, like meat, eggs, and dairy, contain all nine essential amino acids in varying proportions. Animal products are often referred to as "complete proteins." However, the exact amino acid composition can vary depending on the specific type of meat. Eating the carnivore rainbow, or a variety of meat types, during your 30-day carnivore boot camp can help ensure you are optimizing your nutrition. These include:

- **Beef:** Beef is an excellent source of all essential amino acids, with particularly high levels of leucine, lysine, and tryptophan.

- **Chicken:** Chicken also provides all essential amino acids, with higher levels of lysine, methionine, and tryptophan compared to beef.

- **Fish:** Fish is rich in essential amino acids, especially lysine, methionine, and tryptophan.

- **Pork:** Pork is another complete protein source, with balanced amounts of all essential amino acids.

- **Eggs:** Eggs are considered an excellent source of all essential amino acids, providing complete protein in a highly digestible form.

## THE KETO DIET VS. CARNIVORE

How is the carnivore diet different from the keto diet? A ketogenic, or keto, diet adheres to a high-fat, moderate-protein, low-carb macronutrient split. The name of the diet refers to its aim to induce a state of ketosis, where the body primarily burns fat for energy instead of carbohydrates. The benefits of a keto diet have been researched since the 1930s[13] and include weight loss, improved blood sugar

# Benefits of Essential Amino Acids[12]

### Histidine

- Precursor to histamine, which is involved in immune response and neurotransmission
- Supports the maintenance of the myelin sheath, protecting nerve cells

### Isoleucine

- Important for muscle metabolism, growth, and repair
- Involved in energy regulation and glucose uptake into cells
- Supports hemoglobin formation and regulates blood sugar levels

### Leucine

- Stimulates muscle protein synthesis, crucial for muscle growth and repair
- Acts as a signal for muscle protein synthesis, promoting muscle recovery after exercise
- May help regulate blood sugar levels and promote fat loss

### Lysine

- Essential for collagen formation, supporting skin, tendon, and bone health
- Required for calcium absorption and collagen synthesis, important for bone health
- Plays a role in the production of carnitine, which is involved in energy metabolism

### Methionine

- Acts as a precursor for other amino acids and molecules, including cysteine, taurine, and glutathione
- Important for liver function and detoxification processes
- Required for the synthesis of creatine, which plays a role in energy production in muscles

### Phenylalanine

- Precursor to tyrosine, which is essential for the production of neurotransmitters like dopamine, adrenaline, and noradrenaline
- Supports mood regulation, cognitive function, and stress response
- Involved in the synthesis of melanin, the pigment responsible for skin and hair color

### Threonine

- Essential for the formation of structural proteins like collagen and elastin
- Supports immune function and antibody production
- Involved in the synthesis of neurotransmitters and the maintenance of proper nervous system function

### Tryptophan

- Precursor to serotonin, a neurotransmitter that regulates mood, sleep, and appetite
- Supports relaxation and sleep by promoting the production of melatonin
- Plays a role in immune function and helps regulate inflammation

### Valine

- Important for muscle metabolism and tissue repair
- Acts as a source of energy for muscles during exercise
- Supports cognitive function and may help improve endurance and exercise performance

control, enhanced mental clarity and focus, increased energy levels, appetite control and reduced cravings, improved lipid profile, and possible therapeutic benefits for certain conditions like epilepsy and cancer.

Ketogenic macros refer to the macronutrient ratios typically followed in a ketogenic diet.

**FAT: 70–80% of 2,000 calories = 1,400–1,600 calories from fat**

*Since fat provides 9 calories per gram, this equates to 156–178 grams of fat per day.*

**PROTEIN: 20–25% of 2,000 calories = 400–500 calories from protein**

*Since protein provides 4 calories per gram, this equates to 100–125 grams of protein per day.*

**CARBOHYDRATES: 5–10% of 2,000 calories = 100–200 calories from carbohydrates**

*Since carbohydrates also provide 4 calories per gram, this equates to 25–50 grams of carbohydrates per day.*

On the other hand, a carnivore diet is a food source diet, not a macro diet. This means it is not focused on the macronutrient composition of your diet, but rather the nutrition source of your diet. What it does have in common with a keto diet is that meat naturally tends to fall within a ketogenic macro split of 70 to 80 percent of macronutrients coming from fat and 20 to 30 percent from protein.

If you are coming to carnivore from a keto background, you may be surprised that keto macros are *not* the gold standard in the carnivore community. Finding the macro split of protein and fat that works best for you may take some trial and error. It is also highly dependent upon your health goals. Typically, carnivores who are trying to heal fall on the higher end of the fat spectrum (80 percent or more of total calories from fat). Carnivores who are trying to lose weight and build lean muscle mass fall on the higher end of the protein spectrum (30 percent or more of total calories from protein). However, most carnivores find they naturally fall in a 20 to 30 percent protein and 70 to 80 percent fat macro split.

Many carnivores report feeling their best when eating within a ketogenic macro range due to the benefits of ketosis, including accelerated fat loss,[14] reduced inflammation,[15] and therapeutic effects on certain chronic illnesses.[16] Not only do they get all the benefits from nutritionally dense meat, but they also leverage the benefits of an energy-rich macronutrient state. Interestingly, the macros from both the hanging weight (edible meat from) of cows and eggs is 60 percent of the calories from fat and 40 percent from protein. Not coincidentally, there appears to be a trend with long-term carnivores to settle at this macro split. Nature knows what it is doing!

## NUTRIENT DENSITY AND BIOAVAILABILITY: WHY IT MATTERS

Beyond the complete protein profile in meat, there are other vitamins and nutrients that are more bioavailable than they are in plant foods. *Bioavailability* refers to the ability of your body to access and utilize the nutrition in your food. Eating food sources with bioavailable nutrients makes your diet more efficient; you need to eat less food to gain more health benefits than you otherwise would.

**Iron:** Meat, especially red meat, is the best source of heme iron. Heme iron is more easily absorbed by the body than non-heme iron, the form of iron found in plant-based foods. Iron is essential for oxygen transport and delivery to the cells. You would need to consume three times the amount[17] of non-heme as heme iron to reap the same nutritional benefits.

**Vitamin $B_{12}$:** Vitamin $B_{12}$ is essential for blood and nerve cell health, and it also helps make DNA, the genetic material in all of your cells.[18] Vitamin $B_{12}$ is not available in most plant-based foods and therefore must be supplemented by those eating a plant-based diet. A deficiency of $B_{12}$ can lead to symptoms ranging from fatigue to early onset dementia.[19]

**Zinc:** Another mineral abundant in meat is zinc. It's necessary for many functions in the body, including immune function and wound healing. While zinc is available from plant sources, other elements of plants, like phytates and fiber, prevent absorption in the gastrointestinal tract.[20]

**Vitamin A:** Like iron, the form of vitamin A present in meat and plant-based foods differs.[21] In meat, preformed vitamin A is present. In plants, carotenoids, or provitamins, are found. Provitamin A provides the body with everything it needs to synthesize vitamin A, but requires additional processing, making it less efficient than the preformed vitamin A found in meat sources.

## PLANT TOXINS

Plants can't run away. As plants co-evolved with herbivorous and omnivorous creatures, they developed defense mechanisms to being eaten. They do this by way of the toxins present in their leaves, stems, seeds, and roots. While many plant toxins are harmless in small amounts, some can be harmful or toxic to humans and animals if overconsumed.[22] It is important to note that the chemist adage that "the dose makes the poison" is applicable here. This is because the harmful effects you may experience from these toxins is dependent upon the amount that's consumed and your bio-individual resilience to them.

Understanding plant toxins and how each toxin might be impacting your health can help you understand which plants are the most important for you to avoid. While this list isn't comprehensive of all possible plant toxins, their effects, and their sources, it shows that certain plants can be problematic when we consume them as a food source.

**Lectins:** Lectins are a protein found in many plants, including beans, legumes, and the nightshade family. This toxin damages the digestive tract and can trigger autoimmune issues.[23]

Some foods high in lectins: beans, peanuts, whole grains, soybeans, potatoes, tomatoes

**Phytates (Phytic Acid):** Typically found in plant seeds, phytates inhibit the absorption of iron, zinc, copper, magnesium, and calcium.[24]

Some foods high in phytates: beans, seeds, nuts, grains

**Polyphenols:** Polyphenols are often heralded as a huge benefit to eating a plant-based diet. However, polyphenols have also been linked to high blood pressure and thyroid disease.[25] Polyphenols are found in many plants, especially those heralded as "superfoods."

Some foods high in polyphenols: apples, red wine, chocolate, olive oil, turmeric

**Glucosinolates/Sulforaphanes:** This toxin is often found in cruciferous vegetables and has been shown to have toxic effects that block the absorption of iodine[26] and can act as goitrogens (antithyroid agents).

Some foods high in sulforaphane: broccoli, cauliflower, Brussels sprouts, cabbage

**Oxalic Acid:** Oxalic acid, also known as oxalate, is found in many plant foods. Oxalic acids form crystal structures that build up in areas of inflammation in the body, often causing joint pain.[27] Oxalic acid can also interfere with digestion because it acts as an enzyme inhibitor. See page 154 for more on oxalates.

Some foods high in oxalates: beans, berries, chocolate, dark green vegetables, grains

**FODMAP:** FODMAP stands for fermentable oligosaccharides, disaccharides, monosaccharides, and polyols. These are short-chain carbohydrates (sugars) that are poorly digested by the small intestine.[28]

Some foods high in FODMAP: wheat, garlic, onion, fruit, legumes, honey

**Gluten:** Gluten is a widely known glue-like protein found in grains. It is not broken down well by stomach acid, often leading to severe digestive issues as it damages the small intestine.[29]

A food high in gluten: wheat

**Salicylates:** Salicylates are present in virtually all plant foods. In large doses, they cause health issues. But for people who are salicylate intolerant, even small amounts can cause many different issues, including headaches, rashes, GI issues, sinusitis, fatigue, swelling, and the list goes on and on.[30]

Some foods high in salicylates: nearly all plant foods, including coconut, avocado, very dark chocolate

**Pesticides:** Pesticides are chemicals used to deter pest infestation of plant crops. These chemicals are stored in your colon and can slowly poison you. Many of these chemicals impact many systems in the body, including nervous, reproductive, and endocrine functions, and are linked to many chronic illnesses, including cancer,

> ## Finding Your Health Baseline
>
> One of the greatest benefits of eating a carnivore diet is eliminating all the "noise" from your health baseline. By removing excess toxins and chemicals from your diet you can eliminate any symptoms caused by unnatural additions to your diet. Once you understand your health potential, you can better understand how these toxins are contributing to your overall health status so that you can feel empowered to make informed decisions about what you consume.

Alzheimer's disease, mental illness, and autoimmune disease.[31]

Some foods high in pesticides: berries, spinach, kale, nectarines, apples, grapes, cherries, peaches, pears, peppers, celery, tomatoes

**Fructose:** Fructose is sometimes called a "healthy sugar" alternative to glucose; however, there is growing evidence to suggest that fructose has negative impacts on the human body. It may increase the level of small-particle LDL cholesterol, cause visceral fat accumulation, increase cardiovascular disease risk, increase insulin resistance, cause leptin resistance, increase uric acid levels in the body leading to gout and high blood pressure, and cause nonalcoholic fatty liver disease.[32]

Some foods high in fructose: fruits, honey

**Fiber:** Fiber is often lauded as a huge benefit to eating a plant-rich diet. The most often cited benefit of fiber is improved digestion; however, some studies show that fiber damages the intestinal lining and thereby prevents nutrient absorption and increases the body's inflammatory response.[33]

Some foods high in fiber: beans, broccoli, berries, avocados, grain, apples

## THE BENEFITS OF A CARNIVORE DIET

There are many anecdotal benefits to a carnivore diet. The Harvard Carnivore Study,[34] performed in 2020, polled over 2,000 people who had been following a carnivore diet for six months or longer to understand the benefits of eating this way. Both mental and physical health benefits were reported from those following a meat-based way of eating.

Based on my experience as a member of the online carnivore community and as a carnivore coach, the top four benefits people are looking for when starting a carnivore diet are: to lose weight, improve physical health, optimize performance, and boost mental and emotional health.

### Weight Loss

In my experience, this is probably the top reason people decide to pursue a carnivore diet, and with good reason! A carnivore diet can help with weight management by naturally reducing calorie intake, increasing satiety, enhancing fat burning, stabilizing blood sugar, and reducing water retention. All of these mechanisms contribute to easily achieved and maintained weight loss through a carnivore diet.

**Reduced Calorie Intake:** A carnivore diet eliminates high-calorie, processed foods, refined carbohydrates, and sugary snacks commonly found in modern diets. By focusing primarily on animal-based foods, which are more nutrient-dense and satisfying, many people find they naturally consume fewer calories. Excessive calorie intake is one of the main factors in weight gain, so eating an appropriate amount of calories is one of the key components to maintaining a healthy weight.

**Increased Satiety:** Meat and other animal-based foods are naturally high in protein and fat, and therefore tend to be more filling and satiating than carbohydrates. This can help reduce overall calorie intake because animal-based foods reduce or eliminate cravings.

**Enhanced Fat Burning:** Restricting carbohydrate intake forces the body to rely on an alternative fuel source for energy: fat. While some dietary fat will be converted to energy, body fat can also be leveraged for ketogenic energy production. Ketones, produced from oxidizing body fat, can suppress appetite and promote fat loss, further contributing to weight loss on a carnivore diet.

**Blood Sugar Stabilization:** Another benefit to eliminating carbohydrates from the diet is stabilizing blood sugar levels and reducing insulin spikes and crashes. Managing blood sugar helps prevent hunger cravings, reduces the likelihood of snacking, and promotes fat burning, all of which can further support weight loss efforts.

**Water Weight Management:** Carbohydrates can cause the body to retain water, leading to fluctuations in weight. By eliminating carbohydrates through a carnivore way of eating, you may experience a reduction in water weight, which can contribute to initial weight loss.

### Physical Health

Almost all of the Harvard Carnivore Study respondents[35] claimed they were trying a carnivore diet to improve their physical health. For many, nutrition is the most accessible form of health care. We all have to eat, and if we have the privilege of being able to choose healthy food, we can greatly impact our health through our nutritional choices.

Some of the reported health benefits from people who responded to the Harvard Carnivore Study[36] include: improved metabolic health; reduced inflammation and associated symptoms, such as fatigue, hair loss, and joint pain; and allergy relief. The benefits from reducing inflammation and increasing the nutritional content of your diet can translate into improved quality of life by reducing or eliminating symptoms associated with chronic illness. It is important to note that

## Using the Carnivore Diet as an Elimination Protocol

The most powerful use of the carnivore diet is as an elimination protocol. By removing all the excess from your diet and focusing on nutritionally dense food, you can establish a health baseline: an understanding of what your health is like without the confounding factor of inflammation or symptoms caused by your diet. That said, if you pursue carnivore for a significant period of time and still experience chronic health issues, you may need to do more research or consult with experts to see whether there are any treatments that could help you achieve root-cause healing.

while carnivore may help you manage symptoms, it's not a replacement for treating root-cause health issues.

**Improved Metabolic Health:** Some champions of the carnivore diet suggest that it may improve markers of metabolic health, such as insulin sensitivity, blood sugar levels, and lipid profiles. By eliminating carbohydrates and relying primarily on protein and fat for fuel, the diet may help stabilize blood sugar levels and reduce insulin resistance, which are important factors in metabolic health. Eating carnivore may also increase the ratio of HDL, or "good," cholesterol in the body, which can help lower

inflammation and optimize cholesterol functions.[37]

**Reduced Inflammation:** Certain plant toxins may trigger inflammation in some people. By eliminating these compounds from your diet, the carnivore diet may help reduce overall inflammation in your body. Especially for those experiencing chronic inflammation, such as arthritis and autoimmune diseases, a carnivore way of eating may help alleviate symptoms. Allowing chronic inflammation to go unchecked can lead to long-term structural damage, reduced immune function, accelerated aging, and poor mental health outcomes.[38]

**Allergy Relief:** Although most people are familiar with seasonal allergies and fatal food allergies, such as a peanut allergy, few are familiar with the epidemic of non-fatal histamine response[39] to many foods. A nonfatal histamine response is a reaction in the body caused by histamine release, a normal inflammatory response to dietary intolerances and irritants.

A histamine response to foods can result in a plethora of symptoms, including skin reactions and respiratory, gastrointestinal, cardiovascular, neurological, and inflammation symptoms. If you have food sensitivities or allergies to certain plant foods, you may find relief by following a carnivore diet and eliminating gluten, dairy, and various plant proteins.

### Optimize Performance

For people who feel generally healthy and already have their ideal body composition, a carnivore diet can help them reach the next level in their fitness and performance goals.[40] Eating a meat-based diet provides the protein, energy, and nutrients you need to feel your best. When you feel your best, you can perform as the best possible version of you.

Animal products are rich sources of high-quality protein, containing all the essential amino acids in the right proportions for our needs. Protein is essential for muscle repair, growth, and overall tissue maintenance. If you participate in intense physical activities that require muscle repair and growth, a diet rich in animal protein can support your performance by aiding in muscle recovery and strength development.

Carbohydrates cause fluctuations in blood sugar levels, leading to energy crashes and cravings. By primarily consuming meat, which is virtually carbohydrate-free, some people may experience more stable energy levels throughout the day. This stability can be beneficial for maintaining focus and productivity, particularly in tasks requiring sustained mental or physical effort.

Meat is also a dense source of essential vitamins and minerals, such as iron, zinc, vitamin $B_{12}$, and omega-3 fatty acids. These nutrients are crucial for various physiological functions, including oxygen transport, immune function, and cognitive performance. By focusing on meat-based foods, you can ensure you are obtaining these vital nutrients in abundance, potentially enhancing overall health and performance.

## Mental and Emotional Health

Another wonderful benefit of the carnivore diet may be improved mental and emotional health. The Harvard Carnivore Study respondents reported better mental health outcomes than before they started the diet. There are a few different benefits by which carnivore can help improve mental health, including by reducing inflammation, stabilizing blood sugar, eliminating allergens and toxins, and consuming nutrient-dense foods.

**Inflammation Reduction:** Over the past decade or so, chronic inflammation has increasingly been recognized as a significant factor in mental health disorders.[41] Inflammation is associated with a range of conditions, including depression, anxiety, and cognitive decline. Inflammatory processes in the body can trigger immune responses that can result in the release of pro-inflammatory proteins called cytokines. This can lead to neuroinflammation and alterations in neurotransmitter function.

Inflammation can also disrupt normal brain signaling pathways, impair neuroplasticity, and contribute to mood disturbances and cognitive dysfunction. Chronic inflammation can induce oxidative stress, which can damage brain cells and make existing mental health symptoms worse. A carnivore diet may help reduce inflammation and therefore improve mental health outcomes.

**Blood Sugar Stabilization:** Blood sugar has a profound impact on your mental health because it affects your brain function and

## Seed Oils, Inflammation, and Anxiety

Anxiety and anxiety disorder diagnoses appear to be on the rise.[42] While some of the anxiety epidemic may be attributed to our modern stress-filled environment, some of it can be attributed to our modern nutritional practices.[43] Seed oils, the oils extracted from the seeds of various plants, such as sunflower, soybean, canola, and sesame, commonly used for cooking and food processing, may be a contributing factor to anxiety disorders.

Seed oils are highly volatile, meaning they oxidize easily. The processing seeds go through in order to extract their oils results in an unstable cellular structure. The food we eat turns into the building blocks our bodies use to form structures in our bodies.

Our brains are almost pure fat: every single one of our nerves is covered in a fatty, protective layer called a myelin sheath. If we provide our bodies with volatile fats to build structures from, then those structures may be easily compromised. This can lead to inflammation, especially in the brain.

Neuroinflammation is associated with a lot of different negative health effects. In fact, research has shown that changes to brain structures from neuroinflammation may predict anxiety disorder manifestation.[44] Eating structurally stable healthy fats, like omega-3s found in animal products, can prevent neuroinflammation and protect against other causes of neuro- inflammation too![45]

neurotransmitter activity.[46] Changes to your blood sugar levels, especially extreme highs (hyperglycemia) and lows (hypoglycemia), can impact your mood, cognition, and overall mental well-being.

Hypoglycemia can lead to symptoms such as irritability, confusion, difficulty concentrating, and mood swings, as the brain relies heavily on glucose for energy. On the other hand, chronic hyperglycemia, often associated with conditions like type 2 diabetes, has been linked to cognitive decline, depression, anxiety, and an increased risk of neurodegenerative diseases.

Eating a carnivore diet can help stabilize blood sugar levels by producing consistent energy from fat oxidation and supplementing the brain's glucose needs by converting protein to glucose as needed through a process called gluconeogenesis.

**Allergen and Toxin Elimination:** Plant toxins primarily impact physical health. For example, plant proteins like gluten may compromise the integrity of the gut lining, causing issues like leaky gut, preventing absorption of essential nutrients. Lectins bind to vitamins and minerals, also preventing absorption of nutrition. FODMAP and phytates can increase inflammation, leading to neuroinflammation. All to say, negative physical health can impact your mental health because your body is not able to perform as optimally as it otherwise would.

While there is limited research on how plant toxins directly impact mental health, plant toxins like caffeine,[47] nicotine,[48] and opium[49] have known effects on mental activity by stimulating or suppressing neural effects. Future research may reveal more about how plant toxins directly impact our mental health. At the least, eating a carnivore diet supports mental health by eliminating unnecessary toxins that may cause health issues.

**Nutrient Density:** An essential component of optimal mental health is optimal nutrition. As I've said, nutrients are substances found in food that provide energy, support metabolism, and are necessary for various physiological functions. It follows that if your physical health is at its best, your mental health will be too.

## FOOD ADDICTION AND MENTAL HEALTH: HOW CARNIVORE CAN HELP

Food addiction is a complex and controversial topic. It refers to a condition when people have a compulsive relationship with food and exhibit addiction-like behaviors similar to abusing substances like drugs or alcohol. While it is not officially recognized as a diagnosis in the *Diagnostic and Statistical Manual of Mental Disorders* (DSM-5), some researchers and health care professionals believe that certain people can develop addictive-like behaviors toward food, particularly highly processed and palatable foods.[50]

Food addiction, like any other substance addiction, can manifest in different ways, from general overeating to reluctance to give up certain foods. This behavior can be caused by trauma or a family history of addiction. Other disordered eating patterns include binge eating and severe caloric restriction. Many people find healing through a carnivore way of eating, but if you think you might be experiencing disordered eating, help is available at https://www.nationaleatingdisorders.org/help-support. You are not alone.

### Signs of Addiction-Like Food Behaviors[51]

1. **Cravings:** Intense cravings for specific types of foods, often high in sugar, seed oils, or salt.

2. **Loss of control:** Difficulty controlling food intake, leading to episodes of overeating or binge eating.

3. **Continued use despite negative consequences:** Despite experiencing negative physical, emotional, or social consequences due to overeating, people with food addiction may continue to engage in compulsive eating behaviors.

4. **Withdrawal symptoms:** Some people may experience withdrawal symptoms,

such as irritability, anxiety, or cravings when attempting to cut back on certain types of foods, especially those high in sugar or refined carbohydrates.

5. **Preoccupation with food:** Constantly thinking about food, planning meals, or obsessing over food-related activities.

6. **Tolerance:** Over time, people may require larger amounts of food to achieve the same level of satisfaction or pleasure.

7. **Mood modulation:** Using food to cope with negative emotions or to enhance positive feelings.

8. **Secrecy:** Some people experiencing food addiction may hide eating behaviors from others.

## Why Are People Addicted to Food?

People may be susceptible to food addiction behaviors for a variety of reasons. That's because food addiction can affect us physically, mentally, and emotionally.

### The Physical

Food addiction can be used by people to help temporarily overcome physical symptoms, but these quick fixes often come at long-term costs. Carbohydrates are the body's primary source of energy, and consuming them can lead to rapid spikes in blood sugar levels followed by crashes. This cycle can create cravings for more carbohydrates to maintain energy levels and stabilize blood sugar. People may become accustomed to consuming large amounts of carbohydrates in their diets, leading to habitual consumption patterns that are difficult to break.

### The Mental

Your mental state can also be influenced by food addiction, and these short-term coping mechanisms can lead to a lifelong struggle with your relationship to food. Carbohydrates can affect brain chemistry by increasing the production of serotonin, a neurotransmitter that promotes feelings of happiness and well-being. This can create a psychological dependence on carb-rich foods as a way to boost mood. Highly processed and refined carbohydrates (like sugary snacks, pastries, white bread) can activate the brain's reward system, leading to feelings of pleasure and satisfaction. Over time, this can contribute to the development of addictive behaviors toward these foods.

### The Emotional

Finally, food addiction can be a way some people regulate their emotional health, giving them a temporary feeling of pleasure at the possible cost of their long-term health. Processed foods are often readily available, affordable, and heavily marketed, making them convenient choices for many people. Additionally, cultural norms and traditions may emphasize the consumption of carbohydrate-rich foods, further reinforcing their role in diets. Some people turn to carbohydrate-rich comfort foods during times of stress, sadness, or boredom as a way to cope with emotions. This emotional

## Are You a Moderator or an Abstainer?

Even for those not experiencing addictive eating behaviors, it can be helpful to better understand your own behavior patterns when it comes to food. According to author Gretchen Rubin, there seem to be two kinds of people: moderators and abstainers.[52] Moderators are able to eat a bite of something and satisfy their craving. Other people are abstainers knowing that if they tried to eat one bite, they would eat the whole thing.

Moderators tend to maintain a balanced approach. They allow themselves occasional indulgences without strict restrictions because it helps them adhere to their diet by allowing for occasional detours. Moderators don't risk caving into cravings and falling off the wagon. On the other hand, abstainers prefer complete avoidance of certain foods or behaviors they find triggering or addictive. In this case, abstaining is easier than moderation. Abstainers find that clear boundaries provide a sense of control and alleviate the mental burden of decision-making around temptation.

Both approaches have merits, and the most effective strategy often depends on individual behavior patterns. Some people may find that some things can be eaten in moderation while others must be abstained from entirely. Knowing and being honest with yourself about your own behavior is the best way to determine whether you should moderate or abstain in any given situation.

connection to food can contribute to addictive eating patterns.

### How Carnivore Can Help: Eliminating Sugars, Grains, Carbs, and Processed Foods

While a carnivore diet is no replacement for treatment from a health care practitioner or a therapist, it may help curb food addiction. That's because the carnivore diet excludes most carbohydrates and plant-based foods. This can help some people overcome food addiction by eliminating the highly processed and palatable foods that they're used to eating and that may be causing problems.

By removing sources of refined sugars, grains, and other carbohydrates that can trigger cravings and disrupt blood sugar levels, the carnivore diet may reduce the urge to overeat and increase satiation, a feeling of being full. Focusing on nutrient-dense animal foods can also support metabolic health, potentially reducing the desire for frequent snacking or emotional eating.

## YOUR WHY

Whether you are looking to lose weight and/or improve physical, mental, or emotional health, a carnivore way of eating can provide you with a higher baseline of health and performance. Eating a meat-based diet allows you to feel better naturally, with very little extra effort, raising your overall wellness across the board. A carnivore diet allows you to feel better easily so you can spend your extra bandwidth on the things that are most important to you!

Despite all of the evidence that confirms the benefits of eating a carnivore diet, the most important reason for you to pursue this way of eating is because you feel it will improve your life. Identifying your motivations for eating carnivore will help you stay focused on your health goals, even when it is hard, even when it is inconvenient, even when you want to give up.

Challenge yourself here. Don't just put "weight loss" as your goal. You could shave your head and guess what? You'd lose weight! Instead, ask yourself *why* you want to lose weight. Is it to live long enough to meet your great-grandkids? To feel valued and respected? To avoid all the complications related to obesity and obesity-related illnesses? This is a judgment-free zone. If you want to look better naked, let's get you looking better naked! When it comes right down to it, you don't want the thing, you want the feeling you think the thing will give you. You want your *why*.

## Getting to Why

The Five Whys method is a problem-solving technique aimed at identifying the root cause of an issue by asking "why" multiple times. By iteratively probing deeper into the reasons behind a problem, you uncover underlying causes rather than just addressing symptoms. Typically, it involves asking "why" five times to get to the fundamental cause of a problem.

For example, if your goal is to lose weight, you can ask yourself "why?" And perhaps the answer is because you want to become more mobile. "Why?" Because you want to remain active with your future grandkids. "Why?" Because you remember watching your grandparents suffer from obesity and do not want to have the same fate. "Why?" Because you deserve to feel your best through every stage of life.

Each "why" reveals a deeper, more intriguing level to understanding yourself and your goals. It can help you become really clear on what you want in life. And ultimately, it can help you stay on track to your goals.

You can also zero in on your why by asking yourself these four questions:

1. Why do you want your life to be different?

2. What does your future look like if you do nothing to change your current approach?

3. What does your future look like after meeting your goals?

4. How will that future make you feel?

### Is Your Why to Live Pain-Free?

For those who have suffered from chronic pain, the thought of living pain-free might feel like a far-off dream. However, the Harvard Carnivore Study respondents reported time and time again how effective a carnivore way of eating was in helping them manage symptoms, including pain.

While going carnivore may not help you achieve complete, root-cause healing from the pain you are experiencing, it may help alleviate the symptoms enough to give you the time and energy to find a route to complete healing.

### Is Your Why to Age Gracefully?

Another wonderful reason for pursuing carnivore is to age gracefully. As we age, we can become less mobile and more prone to injury. A carnivore diet provides plenty of protein, calcium, and fat to help you stay as stable as possible for as long as possible. Combined with a consistent exercise routine, the carnivore diet can help you live better, longer.

### Is Your Why to Look Good Naked?

Sometimes, we place value judgments on our goals. A goal like "looking good naked" might incur judgment because it feels shallow or selfish. However, a goal that makes you feel your best, and allows you to show up in the world as the best possible version of you, is inherently worthy. Even if other people don't get to see you naked, they will feel the impact that your increased confidence and clarity have on how you interact with the world.

Whatever reason you have for pursuing a carnivore diet, it is worthy of your commitment. You deserve to feel good. You deserve to live an extraordinary life. Your "why" is your guiding light in a storm. Be honest with yourself and what you want, and allow your why to be more important to you than your excuses.

## TRACKING YOUR PROGRESS

Once you understand where you want to go with your carnivore diet, it is important to track your progress to make sure you are staying on the desired path. We discuss tracking more on page 137, after you are past the first thirty transitional days and starting to see results, but it is worth mentioning here, too. While the scale is one way to measure weight loss, including water-weight loss, using antropomorphic measurements like calipers or a scale that incorporates bioelectrical impedence can measure body fat loss. If you are pursuing carnivore for health gains, it can be useful to track your symptoms to measure their improvement over time. Check out the symptom scorecard on page 139.

# 2

# WHAT IS CARNIVORE?

In the wild, hyper-carnivory, as labeled by biologists, is defined as eating 70 percent or more of a total diet from animal sources. Most apex predators eat 100 percent animal products as their only source of nutrition. As apex predators, we can derive optimal nutrition and health benefits by emulating the dietary habits of our ancestors.

**Our evolutionary heritage** comes from tribal hunter-gatherer communities. The key to our evolutionary success lies in the nutrition we used to evolve. With the rise of civilization and plant agriculture, we see the rise of chronic illness and disease. By returning to our ancestral roots, we can leverage the age-old wisdom of our ancestors to achieve better wellness and health.

According to the Harvard Carnivore Study, individuals who have pursued this way of eating have experienced certain health benefits, including weight loss, improved energy, mental clarity, and relief from certain health conditions by reducing inflammation, healing digestive issues, and alleviating symptoms associated with autoimmune conditions.

In my own life, going carnivore helped me resolve a lifetime of physical and mental health issues that held me back from achieving optimal health. By leveraging the carnivore diet as a tool to achieve a new baseline of greater health, many people have also been able to pursue bigger lifestyle and performance goals.

Most definitions of carnivore focus on the inclusion of animal products as the primary food source and generally exclude all plant-based foods, including fruits, vegetables, grains, legumes, nuts, and seeds, and any products made from them. Almost all definitions of carnivore agree on the total elimination of sugars, grains, and seed oils.

Unlike the ketogenic diet, which is clearly defined by its macronutrient composition, the carnivore diet does not have a strict definition. Most adherents to this way of eating agree that a carnivore diet is animal-based and excludes most, if not all, plant-based foods. But, just like the keto diet can be approached in numerous ways.

The carnivore diet can be meat-focused and leverage other nutritional strategies like ketogenic macronutrient ratios, or incorporating intermittent fasting, or restricting your eating window to a limited number of hours per day. Intermittent fasting has been shown to lower inflammation, aid in fat loss, and help the body remove defunct cells through a process called autophagy.[53]

For the purposes of the 30-day carnivore boot camp, you'll be following a carnivore diet by eating the meat you like, can afford, and makes you feel your best. However, I'll explain the different classifications in the next section. Bottom line? It doesn't matter how you or others choose to label your diet; what matters is that you are eating in the best possible way for you and your health goals.

## COMMON APPROACHES TO THE CARNIVORE DIET

Within the carnivore diet community, there are several main approaches to this way of eating. While everyone is passionate about the style of carnivore they use to achieve success, after many years of observing and helping others succeed, I find the best approach to carnivore is the one that's the most accessible and sustainable. That said, different approaches may be a better fit, depending on your health history, your lifestyle, and your goals.

If you are pursuing this way of eating to resolve health issues, taking a more strict approach will be more supportive of your goals. The more toxins and possible inflammatory sources you eliminate, the better you can observe what your health baseline is absent of confounding dietary factors. On the other hand, if you are leveraging carnivore to overcome food addiction tendencies or to lose weight, retaining more variety and novelty in your daily eating will help you better adhere to the diet long term. Allowing flexibility in your diet can make it both fun and accessible, and therefore easier to overcome temptations that may come your way.

In addition to the common approaches, like any community, the carnivore diet is susceptible to trends. In my time in the carnivore space, I have seen high-fat, low-fat, organ-heavy, muscle-meat-only, sardine fasts, macro tracking, extended fasting, and one meal every other day trends come and go and come again. As a long-term veteran carnivore, I can say that the approach that works best for me is to eat the meat I like, can afford, and makes me feel my best!

Keep in mind too, that your diet and goals will evolve over time. As you start your carnivore journey, commit to one approach, and allow it to evolve with your goals over time. Following, you'll find the most common carnivore categories with tips to help you identify the best approach for you!

### Ketovore and Carnivorish

Generally, carnivore is a food-source diet, meaning the emphasis is on the inclusion of animal products and the exclusion of plant products. For those taking a ketovore or carnivorish approach, the emphasis is on the macronutrient ratios to leverage the benefits of ketogenesis, a metabolic state where fat is used for energy rather than carbs.

Typically, people identify with these labels if they track macronutrient ratios to achieve ketogenesis by eating 65 to 70 percent of their calories from fat and 30 to 35 percent of their calories from protein. They also regularly incorporate significant amounts of non-animal products within their diets. Plant toxin–containing foods frequently associated with this way of eating include nuts, berries, avocado, chocolate, and artificial sweeteners.

Ketogenic macronutrient ratios can be supportive of healing autoimmune and gastrointestinal issues and therapeutic for people experiencing seizure disorders.[54] The greater variety of foods in this way of eating allows for more flexibility, especially for people who travel frequently or share meals with people following a more liberal diet. If you want to experience the benefits of ketogenic macronutrient ratios, you can adopt a keto-carnivore diet, meaning ketogenic macros (65 to 70 percent of calories from fat and 30 to 35 percent of calories from protein) without the added plant toxins.

The ketovore way of eating is often the end goal of a carnivore's journey. You may want to use a strict carnivore approach for a period of time to understand your health baseline or to achieve a weight loss goal. Once the purpose of carnivore is achieved, you may want to reintroduce specific, least toxic foods to regain some variety and flexibility in your lifestyle.

## Processed Keto Foods

The ketogenic diet, at its core, is a macronutrient ratio diet. Many processed foods are now being labeled "keto" because they have low net-carbohydrate content. While ketogenic macros have been healing for many, the processed foods associated with this diet come with their own health concerns. Many foods marketed as keto leverage sugar alcohols, which are slowly digested and fermented in the gut, causing gastrointestinal distress for some people.[55] Focus on filling your plate with whole, unprocessed food sources and have a keto treat once in a while.

## Animal-Based

Animal-based is a misleading term for this up-and-coming approach to ancestral eating. Where "plant-based" implies veganism, or the exclusion of all non-plant foods, animal-based is a meat-heavy diet that includes significant amounts of specifically selected, least-toxic plant foods. Additionally, this diet focuses on meat with high-fructose foods like honey and fruit. People who follow this diet theorize that our ancestors ate meat and fruits, when available. They typically include fruit, honey, raw dairy, fatty meat, and organs within their diet.

While more research needs to be completed on ancestral eating practices generally, there is some indication that eating a high-fat diet with a lot of fructose can lead to health issues like fatty liver disease.[56] For those experiencing food addiction, the inclusion of so many high-sugar foods can be triggering. For those with chronic health issues, excess glucose can be inflammatory. However, if your main reason for pursuing a carnivore journey is to improve performance in a high-endurance sport, this way of eating can provide optimal nutrition through meat and extra glucose stores for performance.

Honey raises other questions. While honey is, technically, an animal product in the sense that it is produced by an animal, it is usually excluded from most carnivore diets. Muscle meat is created through the conversion of carbohydrate energy into proteins and fats through the digestive process, literally changing a macronutrient from one form to another.

Honey, on the other hand, is produced from the collection of plants and refining the material by repeated regurgitation into special honey sacs. Eventually, the honey is regurgitated into the honeycomb and dehydrated so that a very refined product remains. The blood sugar spike from consuming refined sugars like honey can cause short-term symptoms like fatigue, mood swings, and long-term health issues like insulin resistance, diabetes, and increased risk of cardiovascular diseases.[57]

## Meat-Only Carnivore or All-Meat Diet

This label is generally used for people who eat all meats, dairy, seafood, and eggs. People who identify as eating this way may choose to incorporate small amounts of plant toxins through seasonings, condiments like mustard or hot sauce, and beverages like coffee or tea.

This is a common approach focused more on the food type—whether it's an animal product—than on the quality of the food source. However, the food source is important. For example, if you have health problems, eating an all-meat diet from high-quality sources like organic, or grass-fed and finished, reduces the load of dietary toxins such as antibiotics or pesticides on the body. This approach is very supportive of healing and helps establish a health baseline. Including dairy, seasonings, and condiments adds variety and greater flexibility to the diet. This is helpful if you frequently dine out, as it can be difficult to find options that adhere to "strict" carnivore guidelines at restaurants.

Don't forget about seafood, which is an excellent way to add a greater variety of flavors and textures to your carnivore diet! Many carnivores neglect adding seafood to their diets because they are so focused on the nutritional density of ruminant meats. However, seafood can provide essential nutrients like iodine and zinc to your diet.

An easy way to incorporate seafood into your 30-day carnivore boot camp is to prepare it as a "side dish" to your meal. For instance, if you prepare burger patties for lunch or dinner, quickly sauté some shrimp in butter and serve them on the side for an easy and delicious way to add more seafood to your everyday meals.

### Primal/Strict/Zero-Carb Carnivore

Carnivores who identify as strict typically do not incorporate any plant toxins, sticking to meats and seafood. While most strict carnivores eliminate dairy, some will include eggs and butter. Egg whites and butter can be inflammatory for some people, while others do not notice an impact. So, if you're trying to go carnivore to achieve a true health baseline absent any toxins, it can be helpful to exclude egg whites. However, if you're using carnivore to achieve a weight loss goal, egg whites are an excellent source of protein, which can help you feel fuller longer.

Meat-only carnivore is ideal for those seeking to understand their health baseline in the absence of dietary toxins. When you remove possible sources of inflammation from plants and dairy, you eliminate toxins, which allows your body to heal more efficiently. Also, if you choose to reintroduce foods one at a time, you can more easily identify which one is impacting your health the most.

However, this way of eating is the most difficult to adhere to if you travel, eat out frequently, or regularly dine with people who have a more liberal diet. If you are using carnivore as a tool to overcome food addiction tendencies, it may be too difficult and discourage you from sticking with it.

### Raw Carnivore

A small set of people are attempting to eat a raw carnivore diet. They adhere to strict carnivore, typically eat a lot of organ meats, and consume raw dairy. The theory is that raw meat is more nutritionally complete. However, in terms of our evolution, humans began to grow larger brains once they started cooking meat. This indicates that the technology of fire, and killing microbes and bacteria through cooking meat, contributed to our success as a species. Cooked meat is nutrient-dense and poses less food-safety risk than consuming raw meats.

### Nose to Tail Carnivore: Organ Meats

Eating nose to tail is typically associated with primal/strict carnivores, who choose to focus on frequently incorporating organ meats into their diet. Organ meats can include the liver, kidneys, and thymus, among others. Organ meats are known for their high vitamin and mineral content, increasing the nutritional load in your diet.

Some in the carnivore community believe that by eating specific organs, you can provide your body with the building blocks for your own organ function. For example, for respiratory health, consuming beef lung may help ensure you are providing your body with all the necessary components of proper lung function. It will be interesting to see whether these theories prove true as more interest grows in ancestral eating practices.

The biofeedback approach is an excellent way to manage incorporating organ meats into your diet. To take this approach, you would eat a sample of a variety of cooked organ meats. In the future, if you crave that organ meat's taste, your body is providing biofeedback that you may benefit from the vitamin and mineral content of that specific organ meat. This can be a helpful way to self-regulate your organ meat consumption. Simply put, if you don't crave it, don't eat it.

If you are looking for an accessible way to include more organ meats in your diet, you can purchase ground meat (typically beef) mixed with organ meats from your butcher or online meat supplier.

With the awareness of the nutrient-dense health benefits of organ meats has come a rise in organ supplements on the market. Supplements are not regulated by the FDA and the actual composition of the organ supplements, especially considering their cost-per-ounce compared to their whole-meat counterparts, has received public scrutiny. For example, If you were to buy liver at the grocery store, typically the cost would be half the price of muscle meat, but organ supplements, compared ounce-to-ounce, can be three or four times the price of muscle meat.

It is not necessary to eat organ meats to be successful on a carnivore diet. But if you have a known vitamin or mineral deficiency, such as low B vitamins or zinc, you may want to consider supplementing appropriate organ meats. Otherwise, it is not recommended to take organ supplements, as there are risks of overconsuming fat-soluble vitamins, such as an overaccumulation of vitamin A, leading to organ

## Too Much of a Good Thing

It is said that the dose makes the poison, and there is such a thing as too much of a good thing. Certain minerals, like potassium, are essential to appropriate electrolyte balance, but consumed to extremes, it creates a risk to heart function. Water-soluble vitamins, like B vitamins, are very difficult to overconsume because they are processed and released through your urinary system. Fat-soluble vitamins, like vitamin A, when overconsumed, are stored in fatty tissues in the body. As they accumulate to excessive levels, they can cause toxic effects, like impaired liver detoxification functions in the body.

damage.[58] If you want to incorporate organ meat but want the convenience of a daily vitamin format, make sure you are purchasing from a reputable source! Look for companies that participate in third-party testing for purity and adhere to Good Manufacturing Practices as established by the Food and Drug Administration.

The carnivore community is filled with companies selling organ supplements. Many long-term carnivores are successful without consuming any organ meats. The only time I recommend using organ supplements is when there is a known vitamin deficiency. Once the deficiency is corrected, you can stop supplementation. For example, liver is a great source of iron and may help balance iron levels in someone who is anemic. However, long-term use may cause vitamin A toxicity. Remember also that supplementing an essential vitamin or mineral may hide the underlying issue causing the deficiency in the first place, hindering long-term healing.

### The Lion Diet

The lion diet is the most restrictive version of carnivore. It's often used as an elimination protocol for severe mental and physical health issues. Lion dieters exclusively eat ruminant muscle meats, water, and salt. Ruminant mammals are those with hooves that chew cud, or regurgitated plant matter, as part of their digestive process. Beef, lamb, goat, venison, and bison are included in this way of eating. Typically, this diet is a temporary measure to jump-start healing by eliminating most possible dietary inflammation sources and providing optimal nutrient density, but if you find you are unable to tolerate a variety of meats over time, you may want to explore possible underlying issues, as this can be a sign of chronic inflammation from underlying illness.

Some who try the lion diet to help manage an autoimmune disorder develop histamine reactions to beef. Beef is often aged to intensify the flavor of the meat before selling it. Microbes in the beef begin to break down tissue, resulting in a more tender steak, but this process also produces histamines that some people may negatively react to. Some online retailers specifically sell unaged beef if histamine reactions are a concern for you. You can find these retailers by searching for low-histamine meat. If you want to eat the lion diet but do not tolerate beef, eating lamb or goat meat is an excellent alternative, as it is less likely to be aged.

Halfway through my own carnivore journey, I developed an intolerance to beef. Whenever I'd eat it, I would have a histamine reaction, resulting in a headache and itchy skin. I realized that my sudden intolerance to beef was due to an underlying health issue. Exposure to an environmental toxin triggered an inflammatory response that increased my histamine reaction to previously neutral foods, like beef. This realization allowed me to address the toxic exposure, treat the inflammation, and achieve root-cause healing. Once I addressed the underlying issue, I was able to eat beef again!

### Ruminant Meats

Ruminant animals have a complicated digestive system optimized for converting toxic plant matter into nutritious and delicious muscle meats. Common ruminant meat sources include beef, lamb, goat, and deer. In the carnivore community, ruminant meats are often glorified as the best food type for carnivores. Ruminant meat is higher in saturated fat, which is incredibly nutritious, as it is a more stable form of fat than volatile seed oils, and it is more effective at building structures, like cell walls, in the human body.[59] It's also an incredible source of many powerful vitamins and minerals, including vitamins A, B, D, E, and K, and minerals like calcium, magnesium, and potassium and omega-3s.

Although the meat from ruminant animals is incredibly nutritious, it's not necessarily better than other meat sources, which also provide a plethora of vitamins and minerals. By eating a variety of meats and leveraging the array of vitamin and mineral composition in each, you are best able to efficiently achieve all micronutrient needs.

### Poultry and Pork

Poultry and pork are both micronutrient-dense meat options for carnivores. Poultry and pork are packed full of over twenty essential vitamins and minerals, including vitamins A, B, D, E, and K, omega-3s, and minerals like calcium, magnesium, and potassium. Pork, especially, contains a lot of B vitamins. For people with hypometabolism who accumulate a lot of lactic acid, pork can help flush out the excess production. Poultry and pork are often more cost-effective than beef, can add variety to your 30-day carnivore boot camp, and are often more accessible while dining out or traveling.

Some people in the carnivore community talk about the polyunsaturated fat content in poultry and pork. Polyunsaturated fats are less structurally stable than saturated fats, making them more susceptible to oxidation, or degradation of their structure. This causes them to expel free radicals, a known inflammatory agent in the human body. However, the absolute amount of polyunsaturated fat content in poultry and pork is still less than what is typically consumed in a standard American diet. The overall fat content in these meats can be lower, so you may want to consider supplementing additional fats, such as tallow, butter, or ghee.

As you embark on your carnivore journey, you can start with the approach that resonates with you. If you are not seeing the results you desire, you can always pivot between the different approaches to carnivore to help you reach your goals. Once you reach your desired goal, whether it is establishing a new health baseline or reaching a weight-loss goal, you can evolve your diet to meet the next iteration of your goal. For many, this means reincorporating a variety of meats, dairy, and sometimes plants, to make the diet more convenient and accessible based on their lifestyle and goals.

### Saturated Fat Is Not the Enemy

Over the past fifty years, the U.S. government has continuously suggested that saturated fat and cholesterol are major factors contributing to heart disease. However, this conclusion was drawn from cherry-picked data that has since been criticized by researchers.[60] Indeed, the government guidelines for 2015 to 2020 removed the recommendation to restrict dietary cholesterol.[61]

Personally, I started my carnivore journey with a meat-only carnivore approach. I leveraged prepared meats, seasonings, and condiments to make the diet super accessible for me. Over my time as a carnivore, I have found that my preference has changed to just meat and salt. I no longer feel the need to add other flavors to my diet.

My diet has also changed as my goals have changed. For example, if I want to reduce inflammation, I eat a higher fat-to-protein ratio to experience ketogenesis benefits and eliminate all dairy and seasonings. It is normal for your diet to evolve over time as your preferences and goals change.

My approach to carnivore is to "do what I have to so I can do what I want to." I eat a meat-based carnivore diet free of condiments and seasonings 90 percent of the time. This helps me maintain my health and fitness goals, which allows me to do the things I want to do—like really cool travel.

When I am traveling, I focus on meat first, but I accept that I will have imperfect options. In this way, eating as "perfectly" as I can when I can allows me the flexibility to eat "imperfectly" in order to have really cool life experiences. All to say, claiming you are a perfect representation of carnivore isn't the end goal; the life you get to lead by eating a carnivore diet the majority of the time is.

## WHAT TO EAT ON A CARNIVORE DIET

Simply put, you should eat animal products. There is some nuance here, and as you dive deeper into your carnivore journey, you may find that you'll need to fine-tune the animal products that are best for your health history and your goals.

Many people starting a new health journey can get stuck in the planning phase. They will research and collect data to design the perfect approach only to find that with each new data point a new rabbit hole of nutritional discovery is unveiled. It can be easy to ruminate on the best meats, best meat sources, best macronutrient composition, and best meal timing.

Don't let perfection be the enemy of the good! The 90 percent benefit you will get from just eating meat as your primary food source will help you achieve your goals much faster than delaying implementation of your new diet until it's perfect. To keep it simple, as you transition into your carnivore way of eating, eat the meat you crave when you crave it.

The carnivore community puts a lot of emphasis on beef, but many successful carnivores start out eating nothing but pork sausages, bacon, and salmon fillets. Different animal products have different nutrition benefits, and one type of meat isn't universally better than another. You may be happiest sticking to one or two food types or "eating the rainbow" by incorporating a variety of animals.

"Eating the rainbow" was a common nutritional narrative in the media when I was growing up. This narrative emphasized the importance of eating a variety of colorful fruits and vegetables, as each color represents a different nutritional composition. For carnivores, by incorporating a variety of meat types, we can include a greater array of vitamins and minerals in our diet without the plant toxins associated with brightly colored foods. In the end, the important thing is to do whatever makes you feel your very best!

## Minerals and Supplementation

An argument you'll commonly hear for the carnivore diet is that it is nutritionally whole, meaning supplementation is not needed. While you can get all of your vitamins, minerals, and essential amino acids through a carnivore way of eating, supplementing your diet can amplify and optimize your results. Consider supplements as nice to have and not necessary to your success at a carnivore diet.

Minerals are essential for many bodily functions.[62] Generally, our environment is much less mineral-dense than it used to be. Mass plant agriculture has replaced the natural life cycle that replenishes soil with minerals. Since our soil contains less minerals, the plants grown on it contain less minerals, and the animals that eat those plants now have less minerals too. We are already starting from a mineral-depleted state.

As essential as minerals are and how depleted our modern diets are of them, it is important to maintain a careful balance. Too much of some minerals can decrease the effectiveness of others. Metal minerals, like iron, copper, and zinc, can be stored in bodily tissues and the overaccumulation of them can lead to undesired symptoms like fatigue, muscle soreness, and gastrointestinal issues. Work with an appropriate

health care provider to assess the mineral content in your bloodwork and supplement as needed.

As I've mentioned before, another option to make sure you have all the minerals you need is to eat the carnivore rainbow. Eating the carnivore rainbow means eating a variety of animal proteins, including ruminant (red) meat, pork, poultry, seafood, dairy, and organ meats. Eating a variety of meats can help you cover more nutritional ground because each meat contains different ratios of vitamins and minerals.

Many minerals are essential for the formation and maintenance of strong bones and teeth. Calcium and phosphorus are vital components to provide strength and structure to bone tissue. Natural sources of calcium include dairy, bone-in seafood like sardines, and bone broth. Phosphorous is easily obtained through meat consumption and typically does not require additional supplementation.

Some minerals are cofactors for enzymes. Enzymes are proteins that facilitate chemical reactions in the body. Minerals like zinc, magnesium, and selenium are cofactors for various enzymes. They are involved in metabolism, DNA synthesis, and antioxidant defense. Zinc is present in red meat but most abundant in shellfish. Pork is rich in magnesium, but it is also present in red meat and seafood. Great sources of selenium include seafood, organ meats, and poultry.

Other minerals, like selenium and copper, contribute to antioxidant enzymes like glutathione. These enzymes are essential for reducing oxidative damage by neutralizing free radicals. A proper balance of these minerals can help reduce inflammation. Organ meats, shellfish, and red meat are excellent sources of copper.

Minerals like selenium and iodine are essential for the synthesis of thyroid hormones. Thyroid hormones regulate metabolism, healing, growth, and energy production. Selenium is abundant in turkey, pork, and cod. Iodine is plentiful in shellfish, dairy, and eggs. Some brands of table salt are also supplemented with iodine. Iodine also helps regulate metabolism, supports the immune system, and can be protective against hair loss. If you are not consuming iodized salt, you may want to consider eating adequate amounts of eggs and seafood or consider supplementing as needed. If you are on thyroid medications, supplementing iodine may counteract their effects. As with all supplements, make sure you discuss them with your doctor before implementing them into your diet.

Some minerals, like calcium, magnesium, and sodium, play essential roles in nerve impulse transmission and neurotransmitter release. These minerals maintain the electrical conductivity of nerve cells, allowing for proper communication between the brain and the rest of the body. Seafood contains some sodium, red meat even less. Salting your food to taste is an excellent way to boost your sodium intake.

Iron is another important mineral, as it is a critical component of hemoglobin. Hemoglobin is the protein in red blood cells that carries oxygen throughout the body, from the lungs to the body's tissues. If you are iron-depleted, oxygen transport and delivery to cells are impaired, leading to fatigue and other symptoms of iron deficiency. Iron is plentiful and bioavailable in most red meat, but especially in liver. You can also cook your food in a cast-iron pan, which will allow trace amounts of iron to fortify the foods you cook in it.

Electrolyte minerals—sodium, potassium, chloride, and magnesium—help regulate fluid balance, nerve function, and muscle contraction. Regulating fluid balance involves maintaining proper hydration levels within cells and in the extracellular space. Electrolytes support proper fluid balance, nerve signaling, muscle function, blood pressure, and pH balance in the body.

However, eating zero carbs can affect your water retention because glucose holds onto water in the cells and therefore your electrolyte balance. Supplementing electrolytes can help your body more quickly adapt to its new hydration state. If you experience symptoms of keto flu, supplementing electrolytes can help alleviate symptoms like muscle soreness and headaches.

Consider adding an electrolyte supplementation product, especially during your transition to a carnivore way of eating. Over time, your body may adapt to your new fluid balance state and less supplementation may be needed. However, if you work out regularly, you may find it helpful to consistently replenish electrolytes daily. Electrolytes help support nerve and muscle function and therefore can improve athletic performance.

## Vitamins and Supplementation

In addition to minerals, supplementing with vitamins can be a supportive, but not necessary, practice in your carnivore way of eating. A meat-based diet provides all the dietary vitamins you need, but if you have concerns, or specific nutritional deficiencies you want to address, it can be helpful to supplement specifically. Working with a provider who can order bloodwork can help you decide whether vitamin supplementation is necessary.

Vitamin C competes with glucose for pathways in the human body because they both use the same protein transporter to enter cells. In the absence of glucose in the diet, much less vitamin C is required to meet your needs. Many long-term carnivores do not supplement with vitamin C and do not appear to show any signs of vitamin C deficiency. However, if you feel that supplementing vitamin C will be beneficial to you, it will not interfere with your new way of eating.

Vitamin D is unique in that it acts more like a hormone than a vitamin in the body. Some studies show that vitamin D produced by the body from exposure to sunlight is superior to vitamin D that is supplemented. I recommend using an app like D Minder to ensure adequate levels of sun exposure. Another excellent source of vitamin D is dairy and cold-water fatty fish.

## Seafood

Seafood is an excellent way to add nutritional variety to a carnivore diet. Fatty, cold-water fish, think SMASH (salmon, mackerel, anchovies, sardines, herring), is typically high in omega-3 fatty acids. Omega-3s act as a powerful antioxidant and can help lower inflammation, giving you greater metabolic resilience. Less inflammation means less energy is needed to manage inflammatory response, freeing up resources to help the body repair and heal.

Seafood is also an excellent source of iodine, which many of us are deficient in. Iodine is an essential mineral the body uses as a component to build hormones, and is especially important to thyroid function. Iodine is a crucial component of the thyroid hormones thyroxine (T4) and triiodothyronine (T3), which regulate metabolism and various physiological functions. People with iodine deficiency may experience a harder time losing weight as their metabolism becomes dysregulated.

Some seafood, like scallops and shrimp, contain trace amounts of carbs. However, it is important to remember that unless you are trying to achieve therapeutic levels of ketosis by eating 60 to 75 percent of calories from fat and 25 to 40 percent of calories from protein, carnivore is a *food-source diet, not a macro-specific diet*, meaning it is focused on eating animal-based foods, not on their macronutrient composition. Even if you are trying to achieve specific macronutrient ratios, the amount of carbs contained in seafood is relatively minimal, and incorporating these foods may still be supportive of your goals. I find shrimp cocktail (without the sugar-laden sauce) is a great appetizer or ready-made snack option when I am on the go!

# Vitamin & Mineral Composition of Proteins

· · · · ·

| per 100g | | Ground Beef | Ground Chicken | Ground Pork | Salmon | Eggs | Milk |
|---|---|---|---|---|---|---|---|
| Calcium, Ca | mg | 24 | 15 | 22 | 12 | 56 | 113 |
| Iron, Fe | mg | 1.64 | 1.26 | 1.29 | 0.8 | 1.75 | 0.03 |
| Magnesium, Mg | mg | 14 | 23 | 24 | 29 | 12 | 10 |
| Phosphorus, P | mg | 132 | 182 | 226 | 200 | 198 | 84 |
| Potassium, K | mg | 218 | 223 | 362 | 490 | 138 | 132 |
| Sodium, Na | mg | 66 | 82 | 73 | 44 | 142 | 43 |
| Zinc, Zn | mg | 3.57 | 1.94 | 3.21 | 0.64 | 1.29 | 0.37 |
| Copper, Cu | mg | 0.05 | 0.066 | 0.044 | 0.25 | 0.072 | 0.025 |
| Manganese, Mn | mg | 0.009 | 0.02 | 0.011 | 0.016 | 0.028 | 0.004 |
| Selenium, Se | µg | 13.5 | 23.9 | 35.4 | 36.5 | 30.7 | 3.7 |
| Vitamin C, total a | mg | 0 | 0 | 0.7 | 0 | 0 | 0 |
| Thiamin | mg | 0.044 | 0.063 | 0.706 | 0.226 | 0.04 | 0.046 |
| Riboflavin | mg | 0.151 | 0.168 | 0.22 | 0.38 | 0.457 | 0.169 |
| Niacin | mg | 3.38 | 8.49 | 4.21 | 7.86 | 0.075 | 0.089 |
| Pantothenic acid | mg | 0.395 | 1.03 | 0.52 | 1.66 | 1.53 | 0.373 |
| Vitamin B-6 | mg | 0.278 | 0.4 | 0.391 | 0.818 | 0.17 | 0.036 |
| Folate, total | µg | 9 | 5 | 6 | 25 | 47 | 5 |
| Folic acid | µg | 0 | 0 | 0 | 0 | 0 | 0 |
| Folate, food | µg | 9 | 5 | 6 | 25 | 47 | 5 |
| Folate, DFE | µg | 9 | 5 | 6 | 25 | 47 | 5 |
| Vitamin B-12 | µg | 2.07 | 0.3 | 0.54 | 3.18 | 0.89 | 0.45 |
| Vitamin A, RAE | µg | 4 | 48 | 2 | 12 | 160 | 46 |
| Retinol | µg | 4 | 48 | 2 | 12 | 160 | 45 |
| Vitamin A, IU | IU | 14 | 161 | 8 | 40 | 540 | 162 |

Source: https://fdc.nal.usda.gov

## Eggs

Eggs are an excellent way to keep carnivore affordable and nutritious. If you are pursuing carnivore to achieve a health baseline, eliminating eggs may be necessary, as egg whites are a common allergen. While eggs are not included in every carnivore diet, they do provide variety and work well as a binder and vehicle for other foods, like butter, within carnivore recipes. If you are leveraging a carnivore diet to achieve a weight-loss or fitness goal, eggs are a cheap and easy way to incorporate more protein.

Eggs are relatively low cost per ounce compared to other meats, even if you choose to purchase the highest quality organic pasture-raised eggs. They are also easily accessible and a versatile workhorse within a carnivore diet.

In terms of vitamin and mineral content, eggs are a rich source of vitamins A, D, and $B_{12}$, riboflavin, and selenium. Eggs also contain a lot of choline, which is important for normal cell function, liver function, and transporting nutrients throughout the body. Egg yolks are an incredible source of omega-3s, so even if you skip egg whites due to histamine considerations, including yolks is an affordable and delicious way to incorporate more nutrition into your diet. But don't throw out the egg whites: you can use them as a skin or hair mask. Egg whites have astringent properties and may help tighten pores and improve skin elasticity when used as a facial mask. As a protein-rich hair mask, egg whites may condition, strengthen, and nourish the hair.

Pasture-raised eggs have been shown to be significantly more nutritious than cage-raised eggs. They typically have a higher vitamin and mineral content as well as a better ratio of omega-3 to omega-6 fatty acids due to the better nutritional profile of grass as compared to feed. While omega-3 and omega-6 are both essential to overall health, too much omega-6 in comparison to omega-3 can lead to chronic inflammation and other adverse health effects. Additionally, many claim pasture-raised eggs have a creamier and richer-tasting yolk. Once you go pasture-raised eggs, you may never go back, and many consider the relatively small price difference totally worth the improved flavor of the eggs.

## Dairy

Dairy refers to animal products derived from mammal milk. Ancestrally, humans began consuming dairy at the point they became pastoral farmers, raising animals on pasture. Interestingly, many nomadic communities today, like the Van Gujjars of the Himalayas, still consume dairy as a regular part of their diet. Cultures that had less experience raising pastured animals have higher rates of lactose intolerance even today!

Most dairy in the United States comes from cows, but it can be sourced from goats, sheep, camels, and buffalo. Butter, cheese, milk, cream, yogurt, and kefir are the most common dairy products in a carnivore diet. The nutritional content varies depending on the format of dairy, but most dairy is a rich source of calcium and vitamins D and $B_{12}$. Vitamin D operates as a hormone that regulates the immune system, and $B_{12}$ is a powerful antioxidant that can help remove oxidative stress and free radicals from the body. Consuming dairy as a part of your carnivore diet is an easy way to incorporate more delicious nutrition.

However, not all carnivores incorporate dairy in their diet. For people establishing a health baseline, eliminating dairy can help get rid of confounding factors like lactose intolerance. If you have a weight-loss goal, removing dairy can be an easy and effective way to reduce calorie consumption.

**Butter:** Butter is an excellent source of butyrate, a short-chain fatty acid that is an essential food source for a healthy microbiome. Butter can be a versatile tool in a carnivore diet. It is a great way to increase the fat ratio in meals with leaner cuts of meat. Frozen butter can be a tasty go-to snack. Butter is also surprisingly easy to travel with if you need to take food on the go.

**Cheese:** Cheese is an excellent source of lots of vitamins and minerals, especially $B_{12}$. Cheese also contains casein, a milk protein that is known in the bodybuilding realm for its slow digestion rate. Casein also activates dopamine receptors the same way addictive substances do. If you are using a carnivore diet to overcome food addiction tendencies, eating cheese instead of carbs when cravings hit can help hack your brain into feeling satisfied as you wean off of highly processed or sugary foods. Cheese as a genre encompasses many different flavors and textures. It is a great

on-the-go snack or meal in a pinch. However, for those pursuing health benefits, it can be helpful to eliminate cheese initially and reintroduce it to test for negative effects once a health baseline has been achieved. If you want to lose weight, eliminating cheese from your diet can remove additional calories.

**Milk and Cream:** Milk and cream are high in calcium, a mineral essential for bone and muscle health. Milk is an easy way to incorporate more calories in your 30-day carnivore boot camp. However, the sugar in milk may prevent you from achieving therapeutic ketosis. A lower-carb alternative to milk is heavy whipping cream mixed with water.

Some people believe that any nutrients to be gained from milk are killed during the pasteurization process. Some people can't tolerate pasteurized milk but don't experience negative reactions to raw milk. If raw milk is your preference, you'll need to seek out sources in your area.

Dairy can be an issue for people with lactose sensitivity or intolerance. Lactose intolerance happens when you are deficient in the digestive enzyme, lactase, necessary to break down lactose, the sugar found in dairy. If you are sensitive to the lactose in cow's milk, then A2 dairy, goat milk, or lactose-free products may be helpful alternatives. A2 dairy refers to dairy sourced from cows selected for their A2 casein milk production. A2 casein has a different protein structure and has been shown to be less allergenic than A1, or typical, casein.

Goat milk is an excellent option for those with lactose intolerance because of the lower lactose content. Goat milk is also high in medium-chain fatty acids, which are more easily absorbed and metabolized by the body. Lactose-free dairy has been processed to remove excess lactose, which makes it easier to digest. Since the sugar content is removed, lactose-free milk is also lower-carb and can be a great option to obtain the vitamin and mineral benefits of dairy if you are pursuing ketogenic macronutrient ratios.

**Yogurt and Kefir:** Finally, yogurt and kefir, especially those containing active cultures, provide healthy bacteria to your gut. These cultured products are naturally processed by bacteria, which consume the lactose, or sugar, as their food source. If you are sensitive to lactose, these foods will not affect you as much as other dairy products. Yogurt and kefir are also an option for those looking to reduce their carb intake.

## WHAT TO DRINK ON A CARNIVORE DIET

Staying well hydrated is key to long-term health and wellness. As you transition to a carnivore way of eating, you may notice that your hydration needs evolve over time. Many new carnivores find that without the excess glucose holding onto water stored in their tissues, they need more water than they did before. Hydration needs will vary widely depending on your health history, your activity levels, and your electrolyte consumption.

## Water

Many people find when they begin this way of eating that they consume more or less water than they have in the past. Many whole plant foods, like fruits, contain a lot of water, so eliminating their consumption can increase your daily water intake requirement. On the other hand, processed foods can have a high sodium content, so eliminating these foods may decrease your daily water intake requirement.

Drinking to satiety is better than forcing yourself to drink. Don't drink more than the recommended eight glasses per day. It will take some time for your body's electrolyte levels to balance out, so drinking more water than you need will delay that process. Your personal hydration requirements will be influenced by your weight, the climate you are in, your activity levels, and other factors. A good rule of thumb is to keep water readily at hand and to drink when you are thirsty or your mouth feels dry.

Remember, though, that not all water is created equal. In the United States, the Environmental Protection Agency (EPA) has standards for the amount of microbes, arsenic, solvents, and pesticides allowed in your drinking water. Additionally, many public water sources in the United States supplement fluoride, which has been shown to contribute to osteoporosis, muscle damage, and fatigue. Filtering or sourcing water from natural formations are alternatives to tap water if these risks concern you.

## Sparkling and Mineral Water

Some carnivores enjoy sparkling or mineral waters for variety. Sparkling water is water that has been aerated with carbon dioxide ($CO_2$), giving it a bubbly, effervescent quality. Some sparkling waters contain natural or artificial flavorings. If you want to establish a true health baseline in the absence of chemicals, it is best to avoid waters that contain added dyes, chemicals, or flavorings.

Plain mineral waters are typically sourced from natural springs and have the added benefit of containing sodium, potassium, and magnesium. These nutrients are depleted in today's soil due to commercial agricultural practices, and some people may find they need to supplement with mineral water to achieve electrolyte balance.

Another option for supplementing electrolytes is with electrolyte powders. These come in a variety of compositions and flavorings. If you find water boring and need more variety to promote water consumption, flavored electrolytes can make it easier to hydrate. However, if you are leveraging the carnivore diet to better understand your health potential—how healthy you can be without the added plant and chemical toxins in your diet—a plain electrolyte powder may be the better option for you.

## Coffee and Tea

Eliminating coffee and tea forever is not required to be successful on a carnivore diet. Coffee and tea are both plant-based drinks that contain plant toxins such as caffeine and polyphenols that may affect certain people. Caffeine is a known stimulant that can raise cortisol, the stress hormone, and lead to adrenal fatigue, causing dependence on caffeine for energy. Polyphenols are sometimes heralded as an antioxidant, but in excess, or in immunocompromised individuals, can increase health risks. For example, flavonoids, one of the polyphenols commonly found in tea, can bind to iron, leading to iron deficiency over time.

The plant toxins found in coffee and tea plants are diluted in water, so you are effectively drinking water steeped in the plants, rather than the plants themselves. For those who need greater variety to enjoy a meat-only diet, drinking coffee and tea can be a powerful tool to remain adherent. On the other hand, if you are pursuing a carnivore diet to achieve optimal health, eliminating all possible confounding factors, like the toxins found in coffee and tea, will reveal your true health baseline.

That said, many long-term carnivores continue to consume coffee and tea with no ill effects. If you're starting carnivore, it's better not to eliminate or reduce your usual caffeine intake until you have fully transitioned to a carnivore way of eating so that you don't have to deal with caffeine withdrawal in the middle of transitioning to your new diet. Still, it is a good idea to complete the full carnivore elimination protocol at some point by removing all possible nutritional sources of toxins so that you can determine if you are negatively impacted by caffeine. You may find that coffee does not negatively impact your health or progress in any way.

If you do want to eliminate or reduce your caffeine intake, it is important to slowly cut caffeine to avoid migraines and adrenal fatigue. An easy way to do this is to replace one-quarter of your typical consumption with decaf for one week. The next week, replace one-half of your typical consumption with decaf. Increase the ratio of decaf to caffeinated beverages week by week until it is fully eliminated from your diet. For myself, I found that reducing my caffeine intake by drinking Swiss-processed decaf was a great balance between drinking the coffee I enjoy while reducing the toxic load. Swiss-processed decaf is soaked in water to remove the caffeine, rather than the chemical rinse used in conventional decaffeination processes.

It's also important to consider the fact that many conventional coffee and tea brands have mold due to inappropriate drying and storage conditions. If you want to continue drinking coffee and tea, there are certified mold-free brands, like Holistic Roasters, Purity Coffee, or Natural Force, that will reduce your mycotoxin, or mold, exposure risk.

### Artificial Sweeteners

As I noted earlier, there are two kinds of people in the world: moderators and abstainers. Moderators can eat a bite of something and satisfy their craving. Abstainers believe that if they eat one bite, they'll eat the whole thing. Some people successfully use artificial sweeteners such as stevia and monk fruit to curb cravings for sweets because they pose a lower health risk. Others find that this triggers further obsession with sugar. Only you know whether you are a moderator or an abstainer when it comes to artificial sweeteners. Ultimately, you may want to consider eliminating artificial sweeteners from your diet to see whether they impact your health at all.

Additionally, artificial sweeteners can have a negative impact on the gut microbiome, the carefully balanced bacterial ecosystem that works symbiotically with our digestive system. If you are using a carnivore way of eating to look and feel your best, artificial sweeteners will likely need to be eliminated to reach your full health potential.

## FOOD SOURCES AND LABELING

When we talk about food sources, we are talking about where your food comes from. In terms of animal agriculture, the source and labeling can be indicative of the quality of nutrition as well as the quality of life the animal experienced. While it is important to consider where your food comes from, do not let the pursuit of perfection keep you from eating the meat you like and can afford. The meat you can afford is still more nutritious than the standard American diet.

There are many different labels used to define the most relevant food sources for a carnivore diet. This knowledge will help you avoid greenwashing messages. Greenwashing is a practice used by some companies to make their products seem more ethical or environmentally friendly than they really are. "Natural" meat has

## The Ethics of Eating Animals

Years before I started eating a carnivore diet, I ate a plant-based diet for ethical reasons. As a kid, I loved animals so much that people asked me if I was a vegetarian, until eventually I became one.

Animal agriculture is misunderstood by mainstream media. The U.S. Department of Agriculture (USDA) is tasked with ensuring that quality of life standards are well regulated. I was shocked when I learned that some videos of horrific animal treatment promoted by PETA were staged,[63] and were therefore irrelevant to my own food consumption.

A common objection to the carnivore diet is the inhumane treatment of animals. However, the quick, controlled slaughter in a meat-processing facility is likely more humane than the death an animal would experience being eaten in the wild or torn up by a combine harvester[64] to harvest plants. No food is death free.

Vegan and vegetarian diets may also ignore the mass amount of ecosystem destruction necessary to sustain plant agriculture. Thankfully, recent increase in awareness of regenerative agriculture, a holistic farming practice that promotes ecosystem health by improving soil fertility, biodiversity, and resilience, is bringing many of these conflicts to light.

no technical definition but sounds more wholesome than the implied "nonnatural" alternative. Informing yourself about what the terms on packaging actually mean and whether or not they hold regulatory weight allows you to make purchasing decisions that best align with your values and goals.

### Conventional

Conventionally raised meat means the animals were likely raised in fields or pastures for most of their life and grain-fed before slaughter. "Conventional" also implies the animal was raised without specific emphasis on pasture or regenerative practices. Conventional meat, due to the inferior feed quality, can have a less ideal nutrient composition, but it is still nutrient dense in comparison to the typical American diet and those nutrients are often more bioavailable[65] than plant sources can provide.

All slaughterhouses, regardless of the meat source they are processing, are held to incredibly high standards, and if meat is rated as USDA, it means that there is a USDA inspector on site to ensure standards are maintained during slaughter and processing. The USDA regulates all aspects of meat processing operations, including sanitation, compliance, humane treatment of animals, and traceability.

Strict sanitation protocols must be followed, including maintaining clean facilities, proper handling of meat and poultry, and implementing Hazard Analysis and Critical Control Point (HACCP) plans. These HACCP plans identify and control potential food safety hazards throughout the production process.

To ensure humane treatment during the entire process, the Humane Methods of Slaughter Act requires that animals be handled and slaughtered in ways that minimize stress. Meat processors are required to establish and maintain documentation that ensures traceability in the event of a food safety recall.

Additionally, in the United States, meat is not allowed to contain antibiotic residue at the time of slaughter. This means the animal (if not labeled "USDA Organic") could have been treated with antibiotics at some point, but there was a suitable withdrawal period to ensure there was no residual antibiotic left in its tissues prior to slaughter. After slaughter, meat is tested by the USDA to confirm the absence of antibiotics and the meat will be removed from the food supply if any is found.

### Organic Meat

"USDA Organic" meat must be raised on organic land with organic non-GMO feed, and the animals must have access to the outdoors. Antibiotics and growth hormones are not allowed. Regulated organic meat also puts an emphasis on animal welfare, meaning the animal must be given exercise, clean water, and preventive medical care in addition to outdoor access. All of these requirements are backed up with traceability; if audited, the rancher and meat processor must be able to prove the standards the animal was raised and slaughtered to.

Since organic meat is less likely to contain toxins such as pesticides and antibiotics, it is an excellent choice if you want to consume organ meats. Some organs process toxins within the body, so while toxins are not stored there, it is best to avoid any toxins, like pesticides, that are being processed at the time of slaughter by eating organic, rather than conventional, organ meat. Due to the overall lower cost of organ meat compared to muscle meat, organic organ meat may be worth the splurge, even if you typically purchase conventionally raised food.

If a product says "organic" without the USDA certification, the animal was not necessarily raised to organic standards. "Organic" is a buzzword within mainstream media, so some companies try to capitalize on the popularity of the word without implementing the practices. The "USDA Organic" label indicates that the product has met their specific requirements.

### Grass Fed and Finished

"Grass-fed" means that the animal was fed grass at some point in its life. Grass contains a wider range of nutrients compared to the grains used in conventional feed and therefore impacts the nutritional profile of the meat. Some people believe that it is a healthier option than conventionally raised animals due to the higher ratio of omega-3 fatty acids in the animal fat. However, the absolute quantity of omega-3 fatty acids is still low compared to other animal sources like salmon.

Most conventionally raised meat has, at some point, been grass-fed. The difference is how the animal is "finished," meaning the food it consumes in the feedlot before slaughter. Conventionally raised meat is given feed, often corn or soy, to help sustain and fatten the animal before being processed. "Grass-finished," on the other hand, means that the animal only ever consumed grasses and forages and was never given feed. Grass-finished meats can also contain higher levels of certain vitamins and antioxidants compared to conventionally raised meat.

Grass-finished does not necessarily mean organic, so if you are looking for non-GMO and hormone-free meat, you will want to purchase organic 100 percent grass-fed and finished meat. Finishing an animal on grass is considered more environmentally friendly because the animal lives in a symbiotic relationship with the grassland ecosystem it consumes. Many carnivores choose to eat grass-fed and finished meat because it is more environmentally friendly than conventionally raised meat.

However, the devil is in the details and the detail you want to look for on meat packaging is "100 percent grass-fed and finished." If the package does not say 100 percent, the implication is that there was some percentage of feed given to the animal that was not grass.

### Free Range

"Free range" is another term commonly used on packaging to indicate an animal's quality of life. However, unlike pasture-raised animals given continuous access to the outdoors, free range is undefined in how much outside time these animals get to experience. In good weather, these animals are given access to the outdoors for a minimum of six hours a day.

### Pasture-Raised

This term typically refers to pork, poultry, and eggs and means that the animal was given continuous and unimpeded access to the outdoors, the ability to graze on pasture, and access to indoor shelter. Pasture-raised is not regulated by the USDA, so look for stamps that say "Certified Humane" or "Animal Welfare Approved" on the packaging.

### Certified Humane

Food with "Certified Humane" labeling indicates that the animals were raised to certain standards of housing, feeding, space, and care. This label is regulated by Certified Humane, a nonprofit organization founded to promote more ethical and sustainable practices in animal agriculture by offering certifications to farmers who raise their animals to the organization's standards.

### Animal Welfare

The "Animal Welfare Approved" label on food is provided by a nonprofit called A Greener World. This labeling indicates animals were raised in environments that prioritize their well-being and humane treatment.

### Regenerative Farming

Another unregulated term, "regenerative farming" typically refers to agricultural practices that focus on improving the environment, soil health, and welfare of animals and plants. These practices leverage ancestral farming strategies to rotate plant growth and animal grazing on the land to create symbiotic ecosystems. The animals fertilize and aerate the soil, creating a nutrient-dense soil for the plants to grow and thrive in. The plants, in turn, grow into nutrient-dense feed for the animals, creating more nutrient-dense meat. Regenerative agricultural practices are gaining greater awareness in the media as they provide a better quality of life for the animals and for the people eating them.

Before the western United States was overtaken by real estate development and conventional farming practices, the American grasslands were described as "swarming" with buffalo by early explorers. These grazing animals lived in symbiotic harmony with the plains where they ate. The buffalo fertilized and aerated the grass, and the grass grew deep roots that nourished the soil.

When these grasslands began to be cleared to grow crops like soybeans and corn, which are plants with shallow roots

## Eat the Meat You Like, Can Afford, and Makes You Feel Your Best

One excuse many people allow themselves to make is telling themselves, "I can't buy the highest quality of meat, so why even bother eating any?" The meat you eat is healthier for you than the processed food in colorful boxes typically stocked on grocery store shelves. Many people experience incredible benefits on a carnivore diet eating exclusively conventionally raised meat. Personally, I have eaten conventionally raised meats for the majority of my carnivore journey. I don't prefer the flavor of grass-finished beef, so I choose to purchase conventionally raised beef instead. Also, I prefer the taste of pasture-raised eggs, chicken, and pork, so I splurge when my budget allows. Generally, I try to purchase the highest quality and most humane meat I can afford. The money I budget toward my monthly grocery bill is an investment in my optimal and future health.

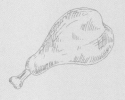

that deplete the nutrition from the soil, the perfect storm was created to result in the Dust Bowl. The Dust Bowl was an ecological disaster in the 1930s, where high winds picked up the now loose and dusty soil, wiping out thousands of acres of crops. "Regenerative agriculture" is not just a buzzword; it is the future of sustainable farming practices.

### Local

Another option to look for is local meat sources. Typically, these meat sources reduce the transportation impact on the animals and reduce the environmental impact of moving them long distances. Buying from local farms or purchasing plants local to the ranchers is a great way to support sustainable agricultural practices.

## WHAT DOES CARNIVORE MEAN TO YOU?

As you can see, there is no one single definition of a carnivore diet. Most people who identify with this way of eating try to align with ancestral eating practices by incorporating more nutrient-dense meat and less modern, processed foods. However, keep in mind that the exact composition of your version of carnivore is going to depend on your health history, your lifestyle, and your goals. In that way, carnivore can be extremely bio-individual and tailored to fit your unique dietary needs.

Many people who have a history of feeling unwell begin a carnivore journey after hearing all the anecdotal stories of healing. If you have suffered from a lifetime of chronic illness, then you may also find healing and relief through this simple way of eating. Unlike other diets geared toward helping people heal that can be complicated and prescriptive, the carnivore diet is an easy and accessible option. When I investigated a ketogenic, autoimmune diet protocol before I found carnivore, I was overwhelmed by the food tracking, specific food lists, and supplement requirements. For those already struggling to feel well, taking the complexity out of the equation by focusing on eating just meat can feel like freedom.

For parents worried about feeding picky children, cooking fun carnivore recipes can add variety and novelty to the diet. For frequent travelers, prepping cooked and dried meats ahead of time, and keeping on-the-go options in your bag, can help you survive any situation. Carnivore is more accessible than many people realize. By keeping an open mind and using the tips in this book, I truly believe that you can succeed at this diet! As a veteran carnivore with many veteran carnivore friends, I have yet to find a lifestyle that cannot accommodate a carnivore way of eating.

If you are concerned about animal welfare, I understand the conflict you might feel in starting a carnivore diet. I was plant-based for three years due to ethical reasons, and during that time, I experienced the worst health of my life. Later, I learned that plant agriculture kills millions (billions, if you count bugs) of animals every year,[66] and that conventional plant agriculture practices are harming the environment by destroying ecosystems and depleting the soil of nutrients. Eating a high-quality nutrient-dense carnivore diet gives me incredible physical and mental health, allowing me to show up as the best version of myself and produce the highest quality of work for the world.

Probably the most important factor in how you approach your 30-day carnivore boot camp is your goals. If you are eating this way to achieve an improved health baseline, then your focus will be on stripping away any possible plant toxins, like seasonings and coffee, and potential sources of inflammation, like dairy and egg whites. To truly drill down on what your possible underlying health issues might be in the absence of dietary toxins, focus on eating meat, salt, and water. If you are eating a carnivore diet to help recover from food addiction eating behaviors, it may be helpful to incorporate more variety through seasonings, condiments, dairy, and eggs to help you feel satiated and increase the accessibility of this way of eating.

Ultimately, the best carnivore diet is going to vary from person to person. Depending on how healthy you are, what resources you have, your dietary preferences, and your goals, your carnivore diet will look different from someone else's. But all carnivore diets should feel abundant—with the knowledge that you are feeding yourself a nutrient-dense, healing diet proven by our ancestors over a millennia to help you evolve into the best possible version of yourself.

# 3

# HOW TO TRANSITION TO A CARNIVORE DIET

The easiest and most sustainable way to transition to a carnivore diet is to eat the meat you crave when you crave it. Your body is going through a transition and for many of us, we are eating nutritionally dense foods for the first time ever in our lives. Placing restrictions on the amount of times that you eat may hinder your progress, trigger cravings, and ultimately lead to a non-carnivore food binge.

**This cannot be stressed enough**—as you transition to a carnivore diet, eat the meat you crave when you crave it. Once you are fully transitioned and have confidence in your new way of eating, then it may be time to consider gearing your diet specifically toward your goals.

## JUMPING VS. WADING INTO THE DIET

Like so many other things in life, getting started is the hardest part. In my experience, most people find this diet through the keto or paleo diet. While some of the principles of those diets apply to carnivore, I like to think of this way of eating as a food-source lifestyle choice.

Some people find they like to slowly transition to carnivore by decreasing their vegetable intake while increasing their meat intake. Others find they like to go cold turkey and dive right in! If you are a toe-dipper, meaning you want to transition slowly to a carnivore way of eating, I strongly recommend eliminating processed seed and vegetable oils, sugar, and any grains from your diet immediately. From there, eliminate plant toxins, starting with any you believe are affecting you the most, one by one until only meat remains. It is important to note that the faster you transition to a carnivore way of eating, the quicker you will start to see the benefits.

Ultimately, the goal is to completely eliminate all plant toxins so that you can truly establish a health baseline for yourself and gain an understanding if there are any underlying issues that may need to be dealt with.

### Jumping Straight In

Jumping straight in, meaning transitioning completely to your version of carnivore overnight, is the ideal way to start. Cutting ties with the way you ate before, fully committing to your diet plan, and accepting the transition from what you used to eat might be uncomfortable at times, but it will expedite the process to feeling successful on the diet.

To let go of your old way of eating, it can be helpful to acknowledge you are choosing a new diet for a limited period of time. The old foods you used to eat will still be waiting for you at the end of 30 days. And who knows? Perhaps those old favorites will not feel as appealing once you establish new health and energy through a carnivore diet.

Committing to your new diet plan becomes a lot easier once you clearly define what that diet looks like for you. Once you decide which variation of carnivore you want to pursue, write out your grocery list and create a meal plan (or use the resources listed later in this chapter for a no-effort-done-for-you plan!). Make sure you have all the tools and resources in place to make executing your new diet plan as easy and fun as possible.

Any time we experience change, we experience discomfort. Even if it is positive, wanted change, we become familiar with our current state. In a way, the known feels safe—it might not be exactly what we want, but at least we know the limitations of this discomfort. Trust me, the health and rejuvenation you can find through a new way of eating may become your new comfort zone before you know it.

### The Top Three Benefits to Jumping Straight In

Jumping straight into your new carnivore way of eating involves an immediate and complete transition to your new dietary approach and can offer many benefits.

**Faster Adaptation:** Instead of gradually phasing out your old dietary habits, and possible inflammatory foods, you have a clean slate. If you immediately eliminate foods that do not align with your new diet and fully embrace your new way of eating, you may adapt more quickly—both physiologically and psychologically.

**Confident Commitment:** Making a clean break from the way you ate before to the way you eat now can reinforce your commitment to the diet and your resolve to successfully complete the 30-day challenge. Setting clear boundaries for yourself from the start may make it easier to resist temptation, overcome cravings, and stay on track. Gradually transitioning to a new diet can create a feeling of ambiguity and wavering that you would not otherwise experience.

**Rapid Results and Feedback:** Jumping straight into your new way of eating can produce faster results. You will experience much faster biofeedback as your body more rapidly adjusts to your new way of eating. Slowly transitioning to a carnivore diet is delaying the physical and psychological effects of your new way of eating. You may notice improved energy levels, mood, digestion, and weight loss within the first couple days or weeks! Noticing improvement quickly creates a feedback loop that allows you to recommit to succeed at your 30-day carnivore diet.

It is important to note that jumping straight into your new dietary approach may not be suitable or sustainable for everyone. It can be challenging and may increase the risk of feelings of deprivation. It's essential to consider your preferences and readiness for change when deciding on the best approach to starting a new diet.

### Wading In

For those who prefer gradually adapting to change, slowly transitioning to carnivore might feel more abundant. Realize, though, that by slowly transitioning, you are delaying the benefits you could experience by transitioning overnight. For those who choose this approach, take this simple three-step process:

1. Eliminate seed oils, sugars, and grains.

2. Start eating more meat.

3. Eliminate plant matter from your diet.

Arguably, the number one change most people living in the modern Western world could do to radically improve their health is to eliminate seed oils, sugars, and grains from their diets. The processing of seed oils results in a volatile and unstable chemical structure that ultimately provides the body with an energy source that releases damaging, inflammatory free radicals.

Sugar is also inflammatory. Every time we consume sugar and spike our glucose, we put our body through another inflammatory cycle. Reducing the number and intensity of glucose spikes throughout the day can eliminate many inflammatory symptoms.

Finally, eliminating plant toxins can remove any extraneous symptoms. If you are pursuing carnivore to establish a new health baseline free from the potential negative impact your diet may have, eliminating plant toxins will help you identify which of your symptoms improve when this food source is removed.

Ultimately, your transition to carnivore is entirely your choice. If you choose to include your "wading in" period in your 30-day timeline, you may be delaying the results you'd see had you done 30 days fully carnivore. Instead, you could qualify your "transitional" period as a pre-30-day preparation for your 30-day carnivore diet.

## STARTING CARNIVORE TO LOSE WEIGHT

When I started the carnivore diet to lose weight, I had no idea how effective it was going to be for my fat loss goals. I had done keto in the past and had weight loss benefits. I thought carnivore would be keto with less meal prep and assumed I would lose weight the same way I had in the past. But while I may have started carnivore for the weight loss benefits, I stayed for the health benefits. As someone who had suffered from mental illness and joint pain for most of my adult life, the results I experienced quickly changed my "why carnivore?" from losing weight to feeling better.

I won't deny that a carnivore diet has made achieving my body composition goals easier. Reducing excess body fat and increasing muscle mass are our two best bets to improving longevity.[67] However, I think focusing your entire carnivore journey on weight loss, and being obsessed with a number on the scale, can make you miss out on all of the additional benefits carnivore can add to your life.

### Counting Calories

That said, when it comes to weight loss, calorie targets are highly specific. They depend on your height, weight, age, gender, activity level, and goals. There is no reason to ask for or chase after someone else's calorie goals. Instead, consider calculating your own. This is my favorite tool: https://criticalcarnivore.netlify.app.

It's important to note that many carnivores find they are able to eat more calories than they did on a standard American diet without increasing body weight. Remember, all calorie recommendations should be used as a guideline and recalibrated depending on your progress toward your goals.

It's important to ensure you are eating enough. Although undereating may seem like a way to reach your goals more quickly, not eating enough may cause long-term health issues as your body consumes muscle tissue to meet energy requirements.

For some people, tracking calories may trigger disordered eating behaviors. For other people, having specific parameters, like a calorie target, can help them stay on track with their nutritional strategy. For most, not tracking calories day to day, but "checking in" with their calorie consumption by tracking a typical day of eating every couple of weeks to ensure they are eating enough, is the most practical approach. You will know which strategy feels best for you, your lifestyle, and your goals.

Eating intuitively is a skill that you can develop by paying close attention to the biofeedback your body provides to you. Whenever you eat, note how you feel. Does eating a higher fat meal make you feel energetic or sluggish? Does adding more salt make you feel more hydrated or thirsty? By listening to your body over time, you will discover the way of eating that makes you feel your best.

## FROM HUNGRY TO SATISFIED

You may notice that you are insatiably hungry when you start eating a carnivore diet. This is a good thing—your body is finally getting the nutrients that it needs! As you continue your carnivore journey, however, you may want to consider the following tips to increase your satiety and improve your hunger signals.

### Use a Smaller Plate

Carnivore foods are inherently more nutrient-dense than any other type of food.

The dish you used to hold your giant salad full of plant toxins is probably disproportionately large compared to the amount of meat you are currently eating. Using an appropriately sized plate, like a dinner plate instead of a cutting board, will help your mind reconcile the amount of food you are actually eating. All of this is to say, pick your plate to match your food, not the other way around.

### Hard/Soft Carnivore Foods

To be absolutely clear, as previously defined in this book, any product that comes from the flesh of an animal—whether it is muscle tissue, skin, or dairy from the animal—is carnivore. However, it can be helpful to think of carnivore foods as "hard" or "soft."

Hard carnivore foods are completely unprocessed and extremely nutrient-dense—meat, eggs, and seafood typically fit into this category. Soft carnivore foods are the less nutritious, fun, carnivore-friendly treats—things like pork rinds, beef jerky, or cheese fit into this category.

Focusing most of your diet on hard carnivore foods provides your body with the most nutrition possible, allowing your body to feel nutritionally satiated. Soft carnivore foods still have their place and can be a helpful tool for carnivores who chronically undereat or are trying to increase their body mass for their health or to achieve a specific body composition goal.

### Eat Protein First

Protein activates your body's satiety signaling mechanisms more quickly than fat does. Protein-rich meat is less calorically dense than fat-rich meat, meaning it takes up greater physical volume. Therefore, it is more physically filling than an equivalent portion of fat. Prioritizing the lean portion of your food before the fat can allow you to feel satisfied faster.

### Eat When You're Hungry

Some carnivores choose to eat earlier in the day while others prefer to eat in the evenings. There are pros and cons to practicing things like intermittent fasting or one meal a day. Fasting may help promote weight loss, but if the time between meals makes you feel hungry, it may leave you vulnerable to cravings or bad binge decisions. (For more on fasting, see page 102.)

*However, and I can't stress this enough, when you are transitioning to a carnivore diet, do not restrict meal timings or frequency.* Eat when you are hungry and have carnivore foods on hand. Don't let yourself become so hungry you succumb to non-carnivore convenience foods or binge behaviors.

As opposed to intermittent fasting, eating frequently is another strategy that may support your goals. Eating frequently can be helpful, especially for people with fast metabolisms, to achieve satiety. There is also evidence that eating more frequently may better stimulate muscle growth.

If you find you naturally graze throughout the day, this meal timing strategy may be more natural for you to adhere to. Some people may find that their meals become less frequent as they adapt to their new way of eating.

## Meal Frequency: OMAD and More

Have you ever heard the term OMAD, OMEOD, or 2MAD and wondered what they mean? One Meal a Day (OMAD), One Meal Every Other Day (OMEOD), and Two Meals a Day (2MAD) are all meal frequency strategies leveraged in the carnivore community.

Some people find they feel most satisfied eating one meal a day (OMAD). Others find one big meal too filling and prefer to eat smaller, more frequent meals throughout the day. You can certainly try different frequency strategies to see which works best for you, your lifestyle, and your goals.

That said, when you are starting out, eat the meat you crave when you crave it. Over time, you might find you naturally fall into a one or two meal a day frequency. OMEOD is a form of extended fasting and is not productive for most people's goals.

### Eating Before Bed

Some new carnivores may find they struggle to stay asleep throughout the night. Eating a small, high-fat snack before bed can support better sleep. Why? If you tolerate dairy well, eating a portion of cheese, which is high in the slow-releasing protein called casein, may help you sleep through the night.

### Eating to Fuel Workouts

Many people find that the carnivore diet gives them more energy to work out. You may notice an initial performance drop as you transition to this way of eating, but over time you should regain and surpass your former capacity. Eating a snack of protein and fat before working out can help fuel your workout, especially if you notice increased fatigue.

## SHOPPING FOR GROCERIES: THE GAME PLAN

Regardless of what carnivore diet you choose, you'll need to shop for food. Depending on the types and sources of meat you prefer to eat, it may influence your shopping patterns, such as if grass-fed or organic meat is a priority to you. Otherwise, most carnivore diets can be easily accommodated by most grocery store offerings.

Most carnivore-friendly foods are going to be in two sections of the store: the fresh meat section and the dairy section. You may need to go down the frozen aisle to pick up burger patties or swing through beverages for sparkling mineral water. However, in general, stick to the perimeter of the store. Remember, you've come to a carnivore diet because it's the best way to use proper nutrition to heal your body from years of metabolic damage, so

## How to Read Nutrition Labels

Food labels can be deceptive. While the information looks accurate, it's not always what it appears to be. Here are a couple of tips to help you navigate the information listed on the nutrition panel of products as required by the FDA.[68]

1. Any claims made on the front of packaging are not regulated and do not reflect accurate nutritional information.

2. The ingredient list is sorted in descending order by amount, meaning the first ingredient is the most prevalent, the next is the second-most, and so on.

3. Not all vitamins and minerals are required to be listed, but companies can choose to list additional ones if they wish.

4. In the United States, calories are listed by serving, not necessarily by package contents.

5. Nutrition labels are allowed to be off by 20 percent, meaning the calories listed may not be an accurate reflection of actual calories consumed—it could be 20 percent more or less of the listed value.

be sure to leverage whole, nutrient-dense foods when you're hungry. Avoiding the center aisles of the store, where the snacks and prepared foods are, will make this easier.

### Alternatives to the Grocery Store

Your regular grocery store is a great place to start to incorporate your new carnivore way of eating into your existing routines. Many carnivores only ever shop at their usual grocery store with great success. There are other options out there, and if you want to look into sourcing different types of meat, it may be helpful to look into these grocery store alternatives.

**Local Farms and Farmers' Markets:** A great way to support your local economy and local farmers is to buy local animal products. You can find these by searching online or meandering through your local farmers' markets. Very often, farmers will let you schedule orders and pick up meat from a designated location, saving you shipping costs!

**Butcher Shops:** As a carnivore, butcher shops feel a bit like a theme park. Butcher shops are typically able to offer a more varied selection of meat and premium cuts. If you are looking for a specific product, you can always ask your butcher if they are able to order it in for you. Other services a butcher can offer are custom trimming, so you can ask for more fat to be left on your meat, or processing meat, meaning you can ask them to slice or grind your meat to your preference.

## Buying in Bulk

One great investment for a carnivore way of eating is a mini or full-size chest freezer. Extra freezer space will allow you to buy and store meat in bulk. Meat in bulk can be purchased at retailers like Sam's Club or Costco or as whole or partial animals straight from a farmer.

**Online Retailers:** There are many online meat retailers out there and each seems to specialize in a different section of the meat market. If you are looking for a to-your-door meat subscription, one option might be ButcherBox, a company that specializes in grass-fed meat subscription boxes. If you want a specific organ meat or type of animal meat, an option might be White Oak Pastures or BillyDoe Meats, which specialize in offering organ meats and low-histamine options.

### Sample Carnivore Grocery List

There is no right or wrong answer to what meat you should purchase week to week. You may be better off nutritionally, though, if you eat the carnivore rainbow. By eating a variety of meats, you're able to get a wider spectrum of nutrients. Keep one of each meat type—ruminant (beef, lamb, bison), seafood, chicken, pork, eggs, and dairy—on hand in case a craving for a category suddenly strikes. You can even program

consistent variety into your meal plan to ensure your nutritional bases are covered. The following lists can help you when you are starting out and unsure what to buy.

## STOCKING YOUR KITCHEN WITH THE RIGHT TOOLS

Now that you know what to buy at the grocery store, it's time to stock your kitchen with the right tools. Making sure your kitchen is stocked with all the right tools will help ensure your success as a carnivore. Your meals may be as simple as buying meat and frying it in a pan, but cooking something so simple requires an emphasis on tools and technique to make sure it is cooked as deliciously as possible.

You may find, in auditing your kitchen, that you already have many of these basic tools listed. There are essential carnivore kitchen tools and then there are "nice to have" carnivore kitchen tools. Focus on acquiring the essentials first if you don't have them already. Then, as you adapt to your new way of eating, consider adding some of the "nice to have" kitchen tools to make preparing meals a breeze.

One of the beautiful things about a carnivore diet is how it eliminates all the clutter from your diet and strips your nutrition down to what is most essential to be well. Meat is simple to prepare and requires minimal tools to achieve a perfectly cooked dish. While it can be easy to fill our kitchens with cool new gadgets or convenience appliances, carnivore keeps it simple, making it easier to stick to this way of eating.

# Sample Carnivore Grocery List

· · · · ·

### Ready to Eat

- ☐ Chicken wings
- ☐ Sashimi
- ☐ Rotisserie chicken
- ☐ Meat and cheese snack packs

### Pantry

- ☐ Salt (I like Redmond Real Salt)
- ☐ Seasonings
- ☐ Jerky and cured sausages
- ☐ Canned chicken, sardines, tuna, and salmon
- ☐ Broth
- ☐ Apple cider vinegar
- ☐ Pork rinds
- ☐ Unflavored hydrolyzed whey protein powder

### Dairy

- ☐ Eggs
- ☐ Butter
- ☐ Cheese
- ☐ Cream cheese
- ☐ Sour cream
- ☐ Plain Greek yogurt
- ☐ Milk
- ☐ Heavy cream

### Deli

- ☐ Sliced meat, such as turkey, ham, beef, and chicken (choose minimally processed options; ideally the ingredient list should contain meat, salt, and water)
- ☐ Sliced cheese

- ☐ Sausages
- ☐ Bacon
- ☐ Canadian bacon

### Frozen

- ☐ Burger patties
- ☐ Fish
- ☐ Cooked shrimp
- ☐ Salmon fillets
- ☐ Ground beef
- ☐ Chicken
- ☐ Pork sausages

### Meat Counter

- ☐ Ground meat, such as beef, chicken, pork, and lamb
- ☐ Steak
- ☐ Beef roast cuts
- ☐ Sausages
- ☐ Chicken thighs or wings
- ☐ Pork chops
- ☐ Pork shoulder

### Snacks

- ☐ Whisps/moon cheese
- ☐ Cheese sticks
- ☐ Deli/lunch meat
- ☐ Pork rinds
- ☐ Precooked bacon or sausage
- ☐ Jerky/beef sticks

## Kitchen Essentials

These kitchen essentials will make your new carnivore way of eating as easy and convenient as possible. Many people may already have these tools, or reasonable alternatives, available in their kitchen. Stocking your kitchen with these resources, if you need them, will help ensure you have no excuse not to adhere to your new way of eating.

**Quality Chef's Knife:** A sharp knife is crucial for cutting meat with precision. Look for a knife that feels weighty and comfortable in your hand. Knives with a full tang, meaning the steel of the blade extends the full length of the handle, provides strength, stability, and better control. Knives with a full tang construction are also generally more durable and well-balanced.

Research brands known for knives with blades that hold their edge well. Most chef's knives are 8 to 10 inches (20 to 25 cm) in length. If you are new to wielding kitchen knives, a shorter blade will help you perform precise cuts. However, if you routinely slice wider cuts of meat, a longer blade will reduce the number of times you have to slice through the same cut.

**Honing Steel:** A honing steel, a long steel or ceramic rod, used before cutting, helps realign the fine edge of the blade, allowing for the sharpest cut possible. Honing maintains the edge of the blade but does not replace regular sharpening. Take your knife to a vendor that can re-edge the blade when you begin to notice that honing your blade no longer results in sharp cuts.

### Cut Against the Grain

Cutting against the grain is a culinary technique that maximizes tenderness and flavor in meat. When you slice perpendicular to the muscle fibers, you shorten them, resulting in the tenderest possible bite. Whether you are cutting a juicy steak or slicing a large roast, using this technique ensures the tastiest possible experience.

**Cutting Board:** Along with a quality chef's knife, a durable, steady cutting board can allow you to make accurate cuts every time. Make sure you have one large enough to accommodate larger cuts of meat. While plastic is convenient because you can put it in the dishwasher, heavy wooden boards are less likely to slide around on the countertop, leading to safer cutting. Cutting boards should be cleaned after every use with hot soapy water and a sanitizing solution (I use a 1:1 water to vinegar mixture), and then rinsed with clean water.

**Meat Thermometer:** A meat thermometer is essential to ensure meat is cooked through and to the desired level of doneness. Digital meat thermometers provide accurate and precise readings. If you cook a lot of roasts, grill, or use a smoker, a digital thermometer with a lead and a built-in alarm that chimes when meat reaches the desired temperature can help you achieve perfectly cooked meat every time.

**Cast-Iron Skillet:** Cast-iron cookware retains heat beautifully and is ideal for searing meat like steaks, burgers, and much, much more. Follow the manufacturer's instructions to "season" the pan before use—typically a process of heating the pan with layers of cooking fat (tallow is the perfect carnivore option for this) to develop a natural nonstick surface on the pan. Start with a regular cast-iron skillet for the most versatility and consider expanding your collection with a grill pan with raised ridges. This mimics the sear lines you would achieve through outdoor grilling.

**Tongs:** The easiest way to flip meat in a pan or on a grill is typically with a pair of tongs because you can firmly grip and control the meat. Long-handled tongs allow for greater reach into a grill or oven without risking burning yourself. Tongs are also helpful when dealing with delicate meats like chicken or fish, allowing you to flip them without piercing the skin and losing all the delicious juices that keep the meat tender and moist.

**Roasting Pan:** The fastest and most hands-off way to cook a lot of meat at once is by roasting it in the oven. A sturdy roasting pan with tall sides allows you to bake or braise meat without worrying about fat or juices spilling over the edge. Roasting pans are excellent for cooking larger cuts of meat like beef roasts as well as greater volumes of meat, like a bunch of juicy, tender chicken thighs.

## Next-Level Kitchen Tools

None of the tools listed below are essential to your new carnivore way of eating. However, they can make cooking meat easier and more convenient. Especially if you are considering pursuing a carnivore diet over a longer period of time, these tools can become a huge convenience to your new nutritional strategy.

**Kitchen Shears:** Kitchen shears can make trimming fat, turning bacon into bits, and snipping the tips off of chicken wings a breeze. Look for a pair that comes apart for easy cleaning. Occasionally honing the blades of your shears will keep them sharp and safer to use.

**Vacuum Sealer:** Buying meat in bulk can be an excellent way to reduce the price-per-pound it takes to feed yourself well. A vacuum sealer helps prevent freezer burn and increases the shelf life of meat stored for longer periods of time.

**Meat Slicer:** Thinly sliced, dehydrated meat is an excellent carnivore snack. Partially freezing pork and beef roasts can make them a lot easier to slice. A meat slicer can help you get thinner, more even cuts.

## Cooking Appliances

Most carnivore cooking is relatively straightforward: prepare meat through slicing and seasoning, and then heat until cooked through. You have a variety of heating options at your disposal when it comes to cooking meat. Most carnivores rely heavily on a stove burner and cast-iron skillet to prepare most of their meals, but you can

## CHEAT SHEET
## Cooking Tools

Having the right tools available can make a huge difference in the efficiency of your cooking and subsequent cleanup. Oh, and on that note, you may want to splurge on the grease-cutting dish soap, as bacon fat is no joke.

### Essentials
- Meat thermometer
- Cast-iron pan
- Spatula
- Tongs
- Whisk
- Roasting pan
- Good chef's knife
- Cutting board
- Slow cooker

### Helpful
- Air fryer
- In-oven thermometer
- Small rack or skewers to dry age in fridge
- Waffle maker
- Mixer
- Blender/food processor/ immersion blender

add variety by incorporating some of these appliances into your cooking regimen.

**Stove Burner/Hot Plate:** A stove burner or hot plate and a cast-iron skillet are all you really need to cook on a carnivore diet. From morning bacon and eggs to lunchtime burgers, to a seared salmon fillet for dinner, a burner and skillet provide the most versatility to your kitchen. If you do not have a stove with a built-in burner, a plug-in electric hot plate can provide all the heat you need with very minimal energy consumption or cleanup required.

**Oven:** Access to an oven helps when it comes to roasting, baking, braising, and dehydrating culinary possibilities. Many large, cheap cuts of meat require longer cooking times to slowly break down the tough connective tissues. The end result is a tender, flavorsome, cost-effective, abundant meal.

**Grill:** An outdoor grill adds variety and new flavors to a carnivore diet. Gas and charcoal grills come in a variety of sizes suited for the outdoor space you have available to you. Grilling can also allow you to cook a lot of meat quickly at once because you are not limited to the surface area available in a skillet. Finally, the controllable temperature variation allows you to cook different types of meat at the same time.

**Air Fryer:** If I had to pick one nonessential item to invest in first, it would be the air fryer. This self-contained cooking appliance makes meal prep and cleanup a breeze. An air fryer is a tiny fan-powered oven that allows you to cook evenly at higher heats for a "fried" effect. Chicken wings are excellent cooked in an air fryer, but you can also cook basic staples like burger patties from frozen in a pinch.

**Slow Cooker:** Similar to oven cooking, a slow cooker allows for long, slow cooking times to break down the connective tissue in tough cuts of meat. Slow cooking is also convenient, hands-off meal prep for a busy schedule. You can put a roast in your slow cooker with a bit of water or broth, allow it to cook on low for 8 hours, and have a hot, delicious meal ready when you come home from work.

**Smoker:** Meat smokers come in many varieties, from the wood smokers you may see at your local barbecue joint to more space-saving options like pellet and electric smokers. Smoking meat can add a great flavor variation from your typical meat preparation methods. Smoked chicken wings, salmon, and even homemade bacon can elevate your weekly essentials to next-level flavor.

## ESSENTIAL CARNIVORE COOKING TECHNIQUES

Before we get into meal prep and actual recipes, let's go over some essential cooking techniques for meat. Learning different ways to cook the same meat can add a level of variety to your menu without having to buy different types of meat.

**Dry Brining/Aging:** Dry brining allows moisture to evaporate from the surface area of the meat, leading to a crispier sear. I like to dry brine less-than-premium steaks

to improve their flavor. Dry a steak using paper towels, salt liberally on both sides, and prop up on a rack or skewers, uncovered, in the fridge for 2 hours to overnight. Pull the steak from the fridge and allow it to come to room temperature before cooking.

**Brining:** Add meat or eggs to a saltwater solution and allow to cure per recipe directions. This process tenderizes meat before cooking. For a fun spin on this process, use the leftover pickle juice from an old jar of pickles to brine chicken wings for at least 2 hours, then dry thoroughly before cooking.

**Poaching:** Bring salted water in a saucepan to a bare simmer, swirl the water with a slotted spoon, and crack an egg into the center. The whirlpool will help the egg white wrap around itself. Allow to simmer to the desired doneness, around 3 minutes for runny yolks. Remove the egg from the simmering water using a slotted spoon, allowing the water to drain off the egg before serving.

## CARNIVORE MEAL PREP AND PLANNING: SIMPLE AND EASY

Now that you what to buy, how to stock your kitchen, and essential cooking techniques, it's time to learn about meal prep and meal plans. You'll quickly find that one of the incredible, and likely unexpected, benefits of eating a carnivore diet is its simplicity. There are a limited number of foods that are typically allowed on a carnivore diet, and a limited number of ways to prepare them. So, you may find that you spend

# Cleaning Tips

It is important to keep your kitchen tools clean and well maintained, so they perform optimally for as long as possible. Cooking only meat may require more attention to fat management than you are used to. With some simple products and techniques, you can keep your kitchen (and your clothes) clean and fat-free!

### Fat Management

Cooking meat renders, or liquefies, the fat content. This liquid fat is culinary gold, but what isn't consumed should be carefully reused or disposed of. Never pour hot fat down drains or pipes. As the fat cools, it will solidify and create clogs in the plumbing. Instead, allow the fat to resolidify before scraping it out of the pan and throwing it away. Another option is to soak up the fat with a grain, like oatmeal, that you can scatter and feed to the birds.

For fat you want to keep, like the drippings from bacon or burgers, strain the fat into a heat-safe airtight jar. This jar can be stored in the fridge and the fat can be reused to cook eggs, chicken, and other leaner cuts of meat.

### Washing Up

You may find your new way of eating creates more fat residue on plates and dishes. Using a dishwashing detergent specifically for grease can help with cleanup. Similarly, adding acid to your dishwasher through citrus additives or vinegar can help remove stubborn baked-on fat from dishes and pans. I like to add a small dish filled with ¼ cup (60 ml) of vinegar to the top rack of my dishwasher every couple of washes to keep my dishes sparkling clean. Check your manufacturer's instructions before adding any acidic additives to your wash.

### Use Dish Soap for Fat Stains on Clothing

The same dish soap that is marvelously effective at cutting through grease in the kitchen also works wonderfully at cutting through grease on your shirt. Instead of purchasing laundry stain- removing products, try a dab of dish soap on stain spots.

less time planning, shopping, and prepping food on a carnivore diet.

One benefit of eating a carnivore diet is not needing to accommodate snacks, because the sustained energy levels achieved through a carnivore way of eating means that three meals a day are all you need to feel satiated. There are still carnivore-friendly snacks if you like, but they are not a necessary part of a successful carnivore diet. Eliminating snacks may eliminate one more level of preparation and administration in your life.

If you want to keep this way of eating simple, you can eat 1.5 to 2 pounds (680 to 910 g) of fatty meat until satiated every day. If you crave variety and enjoy following a done-for-you plan, use the meal plan and recipes below for easy and delicious carnivore meals.

### Meal Prep Strategy

Making your new diet as easy as possible makes sticking to it a breeze. Prepare food ahead of time so that you always have healthy options ready. For the meals or days you have more time, cooking a fun and fresh recipe can be a great way to enjoy novelty and variety. Another way to keep this diet easy is to keep quick-cook options like salmon or beef burger patties in your freezer. You can throw these in the air fryer for your dinner after a busy day of chasing your dreams.

Prep three days of food at a time. After this time period, the risk of food poisoning from bacteria that may have attached itself to the exterior of your meat increases. Also, who wants to eat four-day-old leftovers? *Ew*.

### Work Meals

For work options, it may be best to consider prepped options like meatballs, sausages, meat bars, and burger patties that you can reheat. Packing cans of chicken or tuna can be a shelf-stable option if you need an emergency food source. Using sugar-free condiments like mustard or hot sauce can help if you struggle with the taste of reheated leftovers. Pack your own salt if you want to adjust the seasoning.

### Sample Meal Plan

The sample meal plan includes recipes as well as easy-to-prepare meals, like cooking up ground beef burger patties in an air fryer, skillet, or on the grill, and covering them with cheese!

Depending on your preference for variety or simplicity, you may want to include more or less recipes in your actual diet. Many people enjoy the simplicity of cooking meat, salting it to taste, and eating it, while others prefer the fun and variety carnivore recipes can provide!

The servings provided in this sample meal plan are indicated, but please revisit the information on page 53 to determine how much meat to eat and which ingredients are most supportive of your goals.

# 7-DAY MEAL PLAN

## SUNDAY

- ✓ **BREAKFAST**
  Easy Cheesy Breakfast Taco (page 73)
- ✓ **LUNCH**
  Oven-Baked Salmon Bites (page 80)
- ✓ **DINNER**
  Chicken Cordon Bleu Loaf (page 83)

## MONDAY

- ✓ **BREAKFAST**
  Easy Cheesy Breakfast Taco (page 73)
- ✓ **LUNCH**
  Prep-Friendly Pork Enchiladas (page 81)
- ✓ **DINNER**
  Air-Fryer Steak Bites (page 82)

## TUESDAY

- ✓ **BREAKFAST**
  Make-Ahead Meaty Breakfast Muffins (page 74)
- ✓ **LUNCH**
  Cooked Ground Beef Burger Patties with Cheese (page 87)
- ✓ **DINNER**
  Chicken Cordon Bleu Loaf (page 83)

## WEDNESDAY

- ✓ **BREAKFAST**
  Make-Ahead Meaty Breakfast Muffins (page 74)
- ✓ **LUNCH**
  Prep-Friendly Pork Enchiladas (page 81)
- ✓ **DINNER**
  Cooked Ground Beef Burger Patties with Cheese (page 87)

## THURSDAY

- ✓ **BREAKFAST**
  Make-Ahead Meaty Breakfast Muffins (page 74)
- ✓ **LUNCH**
  Cooked Ground Beef Burger Patties with Cheese (page 87)
- ✓ **DINNER**
  Chicken Cordon Bleu Loaf (page 83)

## FRIDAY

- ✓ **BREAKFAST**
  Make-Ahead Meaty Breakfast Muffins (page 74)
- ✓ **LUNCH**
  Prep-Friendly Pork Enchiladas (page 81)
- ✓ **DINNER**
  Cooked Ground Beef Burger Patties with Cheese (page 87)

## SATURDAY

- ✓ **BREAKFAST**
  Easy Cheesy Breakfast Taco (page 73)
- ✓ **LUNCH**
  Prep-Friendly Pork Enchiladas (page 81)
- ✓ **DINNER**
  Air-Fryer Steak Bites (page 82)

— APPETIZERS / SNACKS —

# CHARCUTERIE BOARD

FOR 2–9 PEOPLE: include 2 cheeses (one soft option, one hard option),
1 meat, 1 cracker alternative, 1 spread

FOR 10–20 PEOPLE: include 4 cheeses (two soft options, two hard options),
2 meats, 2 cracker alternatives, 1 spread

*A charcuterie board is a versatile appetizer or snack to enjoy solo or to share. While a charcuterie board typically incorporates meats and cheeses, non-carnivore versions often include crackers, fruits, and spreads. Building a carnivore charcuterie board is a fun way to share your new way of eating with friends and family at events!*

**MEAT OPTIONS**
Prosciutto
Salami
Chorizo
Capicola (Coppa)
Pepperoni
Soppressata

**CHEESE OPTIONS**
**Soft Cheeses**
Brie
Camembert
Goat cheese
Cream cheese
Mascarpone

**Hard Cheeses**
Cheddar
Parmesan
Gouda
Manchego
Gruyere

**CRACKER ALTERNATIVES**
Parmesan Crisps
    (see page 70)
Dehydrated meat chips
Chicken tortilla chips
Crispy cooked bacon
Pepperoni chips

**SPREADS**
Roasted Bone Marrow
Sour cream or Greek yogurt
Whipped butter or brown butter
Pâté

**PEPPERONI CHIPS**
Slice store-bought pepperoni and place on a microwave-safe plate lined with paper towel. Microwave for 15 seconds, then flip the slices and microwave for 15 seconds more, or until crisp.

**CHICKEN TORTILLA CHIPS**
Slice very thin pieces of chicken into triangles. Set an air fryer to 450°F (232°C). Air fry the chicken triangles for 2 minutes.

# CARNIVORE FLATBREAD

SERVES 2 TO 4

1 large egg white or 42 g
of carton egg whites

¼ cup (60 g) cream cheese,
softened

¼ cup (30 g) grated Parmesan
cheese

**TOPPING SUGGESTIONS**
Prosciutto
Ricotta cheese

Preheat the oven to 350°F (176°C).

Prepare a loaf pan by lining it with parchment paper, ensuring there's enough excess for easy removal later.

In a small mixing bowl, whip the egg whites until they form stiff peaks.

In a medium bowl, whip the softened cream cheese until smooth and creamy.

Gently fold the whipped egg whites into the cream cheese, being careful not to deflate the mixture.

Once combined, gently fold in the Parmesan cheese.

Spread the mixture evenly into the prepared loaf pan.

Bake for approximately 20 minutes, or until the top is lightly golden.

Once baked, turn off the oven and crack the door open to allow the flatbread to cool gradually for about 10 minutes.

Remove the flatbread from the oven and carefully lift it out of the loaf pan using the parchment paper as handles.

Add your desired toppings, such as spreading ricotta cheese and layering prosciutto slices, then serve.

# DEHYDRATED MEAT

SERVES 4

1 pound (454 g) beef, pork, or chicken, thinly sliced or shaved
Salt, to taste

Preheat the oven to 175°F (79°C).

Remove any excess moisture from the shaved meat by laying it on a paper towel and patting dry.

Prepared a baking sheet lined with parchment paper. Spread the meat in a single layer on the sheet.

Salt the meat liberally.

Place the baking sheet into the oven and dehydrate for 5 hours. Crack the oven door every hour or so to allow excess moisture to escape.

Once the meat is crisp, remove it from the oven and allow it to cool on the baking sheet.

Store in a sealed container in a cool, dry place for up to 3 days.

— APPETIZERS / SNACKS —

# CHICKEN LIVER PÂTÉ

SERVES 10

2 tablespoons (25 g) duck fat or lard

1 pound (454 g) chicken or duck liver, chopped

6 tablespoons (85 g) unsalted butter, softened

Salt, to taste

In a skillet over medium heat, warm the duck fat or lard.

Add the liver and sauté until it's cooked through but still slightly pink in the center, 5 to 7 minutes. Be cautious not to overcook, as it may lead to a grainy texture.

Transfer the cooked liver to a food processor or blender. Add the softened butter and salt. Blend until smooth and creamy. If necessary, scrape down the sides of the blender or processor to ensure thorough mixing.

Spoon the pâté mixture into a jar or ramekin and tap it gently on the counter to remove any air bubbles.

In a small saucepan over low heat, melt the remaining butter until clarified. Pour the melted butter over the pâté, ensuring it completely covers the surface to create a seal. This helps preserve the pâté and prevents it from changing color due to oxidation.

Allow the pâté to cool to room temperature, then cover it with a lid or plastic wrap and refrigerate for at least 4 hours, preferably overnight. This allows the flavors to meld together.

Store in a sealed container in the refrigerator for up to 5 days.

# PARMESAN CRISPS

SERVES 4

**1 cup (100 g) grated Parmesan cheese**

Preheat the oven to 350°F (176°C).

Line a baking sheet with parchment paper or a silicone baking mat.

Pile tablespoon-sized mounds of grated Parmesan cheese onto the baking sheet, leaving a 2-inch (5 cm) space between each mound.

Gently flatten each mound into an even disc.

Bake for 5 to 7 minutes, or until the edges of the crisps are golden brown.

Remove from the pan and place onto a cooling rack. Allow to cool until firm.

Store in a sealed container in a cool, dry place for up to 3 days.

— APPETIZERS / SNACKS —

# SHRIMP COCKTAIL

### SERVES 2

1 lemon, sliced (optional)

1 pound (454 g) large shrimp, peeled and deveined, with the tails kept intact

Prepare a large bowl by filling it halfway with a 50/50 water and ice mixture.

Over high heat, bring a large pot of water to a boil. Add the lemon slices, if using.

Add the shrimp to the pot and cook for 2 to 3 minutes until pink and cooked through.

With a slotted spoon, transfer the cooked shrimp to the bowl of ice water, which will stop the cooking process.

Once the shrimp are cooled, drain the water from the bowl and place the shrimp onto paper towels, patting them dry.

Enjoy the shrimp immediately, or serve them on a bed of ice.

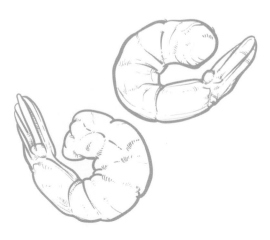

— APPETIZERS / SNACKS —

# SMOKED SALMON ROLL-UPS

## SERVES 1

4 ounces (112 g) smoked salmon slices

½ cup (115 g) cream cheese, softened

On a clean work surface, lay out the smoked salmon slices.

Spread a thin layer of cream cheese evenly over one slice and gently roll up into a tight roll. Repeat with the remaining salmon slices.

Use a sharp knife to slice each roll into 1-inch (2.5 cm) thick pieces.

Arrange the smoked salmon roll-ups on a serving platter and enjoy!

— BREAKFAST —

# EASY CHEESY BREAKFAST TACO

MAKES 1 SERVING

2 slices bacon

1 ounce (25 g) cheese, shredded

2 eggs

Salt, to taste

Fry the bacon in a skillet over medium heat until crispy, remove from the pan, and set aside, leaving the residual bacon fat in the pan.

Sprinkle the shredded cheese in an even layer on the bottom of the pan and fry until bubbling.

Crack the eggs onto the cheese, season with salt to taste, and immediately cover with a lid.

Once eggs are cooked to your desired doneness, cover one side with the cooked bacon, so that you can fold the other half over the bacon to create a taco.

NOTE: Any shredded cheese can be used in this recipe. Some tested favorites include cheddar, pepper Jack, and Colby Jack!

# MAKE-AHEAD MEATY BREAKFAST MUFFINS

## MAKES 4 MUFFINS

Butter, unsalted

2 slices bacon, chopped

4.5 ounces (125 g)
   ground beef

4 eggs

Salt, to taste

Preheat the oven to 350°F (180°C).

Prepare a bain marie (hot water bath) by filling a pan large enough for the muffin tin to rest in with enough water to reach halfway up the outside of the muffin tin. Grease 4 wells of the muffin tin with butter.

Fry the chopped bacon in a skillet over medium heat until crispy. Once cooked, scoot the bacon to the side and cook the ground beef in the residual bacon fat until cooked through.

In a separate bowl, beat the eggs until well combined. Add the beef, bacon, and salt to the egg mixture, stirring until combined. Pour the mixture into the prepared muffin tin. Place the muffin tin in the bain marie.

Bake for 15 to 18 minutes, or until the eggs are set and do not wiggle when you shake the pan gently. Carefully remove the bain marie from the oven, remove the muffin tin from the bain marie, and let cool.

— BREAKFAST —

# DEVILED EGGS

MAKES 12 DEVILED EGGS

6 hard-boiled eggs, shells removed
¼ cup (60 g) Greek yogurt
1 teaspoon white vinegar
1 teaspoon yellow mustard (optional)
⅛ teaspoon salt

Slice the hard-boiled eggs in half lengthwise and carefully remove the yolks, placing them in a medium-size mixing bowl. Place the whites aside, hollowed-out space facing up.

To the bowl, add the Greek yogurt, white vinegar, yellow mustard (if using), and salt.

Using a mixer or a fork, blend the ingredients together until smooth and well combined.

Spoon the creamy mixture into the hollowed egg whites, distributing it evenly among the egg halves.

Arrange the deviled eggs on a serving platter and refrigerate for at least 30 minutes before serving chilled.

— BREAKFAST —

# FRENCH SLOW SCRAMBLE (SLUTTY EGGS)

### SERVES 1

*These eggs were introduced to me through the Egg Slut restaurant chain, so I jokingly named them "slutty eggs." The name stuck and they are still known as such in certain carnivore online communities to this day. They are technically a French soft scramble, cooked in a pan rather than the traditional bain marie.*

**4 large eggs**
**2 tablespoons (28 g) unsalted butter**
**Salt, to taste**

Crack the eggs into a medium skillet over medium-low heat. Add the butter.

Using a whisk, break the yolks and whisk together the eggs and butter continuously. As the butter melts, it will emulsify with eggs to form a homogenous mixture.

When the eggs have thickened somewhat but are still slightly runny, remove the skillet from the heat while continuing to whisk. The residual heat will continue to cook the eggs.

Once the eggs are creamy and soft, but not runny, transfer them to a plate.

Salt to taste and enjoy!

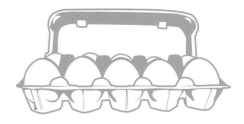

— BREAKFAST —

# BREAKFAST CASSEROLE

SERVES 6

Butter, unsalted
1 pound (454 g) ground
　　sausage
8 slices bacon, chopped
6 large eggs
1 cup (240 ml) heavy cream
1 cup (120 g) shredded ched-
　　dar cheese
Salt, to taste

**Optional toppings**
Chopped green onions
Diced tomatoes
Salsa

Preheat the oven to 350°F (176°C).

Grease a 9 × 13-inch (23 × 33 cm) baking dish with butter.

In a medium skillet over medium heat, add the ground sausage, breaking apart with a spatula or wooden spoon until cooked through.

Once cooked, remove the sausage from the pan and drain on a plate lined with paper towels.

In the same pan over medium heat, cook the bacon until cooked through and crispy. Drain the bacon on the same plate as the sausage.

In a large mixing bowl, whisk together the eggs and heavy cream until well combined. Season with salt to taste.

Stir in the cheddar cheese, cooked sausage, and cooked bacon, then pour it into the prepared baking dish, spreading it out evenly with a spatula.

Place the baking dish into the preheated oven and bake for 25 to 30 minutes, or until the eggs are set and the top is golden brown.

Remove the casserole from the oven and let it cool for a few minutes before slicing.

— BREAKFAST —

# EGG WRAP BURRITO

## SERVES 1

1 egg
Pat of unsalted butter
Sour cream (optional)

**Filling suggestions**
Scrambled eggs
Cooked sausage
Cooked bacon

In a small mixing bowl, crack and beat the egg until the white and yolk are fully combined.

Pour the egg into a 12-inch (30 cm) skillet over medium heat and cook in a single thin layer for about 30 seconds, then flip the egg over, keeping the circle as intact as possible. Cook on the other side for another 30 seconds, or until the egg is completely set. This will be your wrap.

Carefully move the egg wrap onto a plate or cutting board.

Place your desired fillings, such as scrambled eggs, cooked sausage, or cooked bacon, in a line in the center of the wrap.

Fold the ends of the wrap over the filling, then fold in the sides, until the filling is completely encapsulated by the wrap.

Add a small amount of butter to the pan over medium heat, and place the folded wrap into the pan, frying on each side for 30 seconds or until crisp.

Remove from the heat onto a serving plate and enjoy with a dollop of sour cream, if desired.

— BREAKFAST —

# BREAKFAST SCRAMBLE

SERVES 2

6 large eggs
¼ cup (60 ml) heavy cream
Salt, to taste
4 slices bacon, chopped
½ pound (225 g) ground
    sausage
1 cup (120 g) shredded
    cheddar cheese

In a large mixing bowl, whisk together the eggs and heavy cream until well combined. Season with salt to taste.

Heat a large skillet over medium heat and add the chopped bacon. Cook until the bacon is crispy, then remove it from the skillet and set it aside on a paper towel–lined plate.

In the same skillet, add the ground sausage and cook until browned and cooked through, breaking it up into smaller pieces with a spatula.

Once the sausage is cooked, reduce the heat to medium-low and pour the egg mixture into the skillet.

Cook the eggs, stirring gently with a spatula, until they begin to set but are still slightly runny.

Sprinkle the shredded cheddar cheese over the eggs, along with the cooked bacon.

Continue cooking the eggs, stirring occasionally, until the cheese is melted and the eggs are cooked to your desired consistency.

Divide the eggs between two plates or bowls and enjoy.

— LUNCH —

# OVEN-BAKED SALMON BITES

MAKES 1 POUND (455 G)

Leftover bacon fat or
    unsalted butter
1 pound (455 g) salmon,
    defrosted if frozen
Salt, to taste
Cream cheese or sour cream,
    for serving (optional)

Preheat the oven to 375°F (190°C).

Add enough bacon fat or butter to coat the bottom of a
9 x 13-inch (23 x 33-cm) baking dish and place on the
middle rack of the oven while the oven is preheating.

Cut the salmon into 1-inch (2.5 cm) cubes and season with
salt to taste.

Remove the preheated pan from the oven and add the
salmon bites, skin side down. Bake for 10 to 12 minutes,
or until the salmon is cooked through.

Serve with cream cheese or sour cream, if desired.

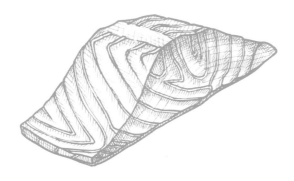

# PREP-FRIENDLY PORK ENCHILADAS

MAKES 9 ENCHILADAS, OR 3 SERVINGS

**For the Tortillas**

8 ounces (250 g) ground chicken or chopped skinless, boneless chicken breast

4 egg whites or ½ cup (120 ml) egg whites from a carton

2 eggs

¼ cup (60 ml) water

Salt, to taste

Butter, unsalted

**For the Enchiladas**

2 pounds (910 g) pork shoulder or chuck roast

Salt, to taste

1 cup (240 ml) beef or chicken broth

Splash of apple cider vinegar

Seasonings of choice, such as 1 teaspoon each cumin, garlic powder, oregano, and cayenne (optional)

½ cup (120 g) sour cream

½ cup (120 g) cream cheese

1 cup (120 g) shredded Colby Jack cheese, divided

To make the tortillas, place the chicken, egg whites, eggs, water, and salt to taste in a food processor or blender and process until they combine into a thin batter.

Butter a skillet and place over medium heat. Pour the batter into the pan, carefully swirling to spread the batter in an even circle. Cook for 2 minutes on each side and remove from the pan.

Continue cooking tortillas until the entirety of the batter has been used. You should get 9 to 12 tortillas total, depending on your pan size.

To make the enchiladas, place the pork shoulder and salt to taste in a slow cooker and cook on low for 8 to 10 hours. Remove from the slow cooker to a large bowl, leaving the liquid in the slow cooker. Let the meat cool slightly, then shred finely with two forks.

Pour the roast drippings into a saucepan, add the broth, a splash of apple cider vinegar, and seasonings as desired and cook over medium heat until the liquid is reduced by half.

In a separate bowl, mix together the sour cream, cream cheese, and ¾ cup shredded cheese. Set aside.

Preheat the oven to 350°F (180°C). Grease a 9 x 13-inch (23 x 33-cm) baking dish.

Fill the prepared tortillas with ¼ cup (60 g) of the shredded pork and ¼ cup (60 g) of the cheese mixture.

Wrap the tortilla around the filling tightly and pack into the prepared pan. You should be able to create 9 to 12 enchiladas, depending on the size of pan used to create the tortillas.

Top the enchiladas with any remaining cheese mixture and the prepared sauce, and then sprinkle the reserved Colby Jack cheese on top. Cover the pan tightly with foil.

Bake for 25 to 30 minutes, until the cheese has melted and the sauce is bubbling.

Remove the foil, turn the oven to broil, and broil for 5 minutes for an extra toasty cheese topping.

— DINNER —

# AIR-FRYER STEAK BITES

MAKES 1 POUND (455 G)

1 pound (455 g) rib-eye or
   New York strip steak
Salt, to taste

Preheat the air fryer to 390°F (199°C) for 3 minutes.

Cut the steak into 2-inch (5 cm) cubes. Sprinkle with salt.

Place in the air fryer and cook for 10 to 12 minutes, tossing the pieces around halfway through the cooking time.

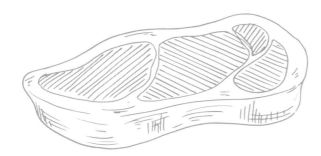

— DINNER —

# CHICKEN CORDON BLEU LOAF

MAKES 1.5 POUNDS (680 G), OR 6 SERVINGS

Butter, unsalted

1 pound (455 g) ground chicken

Salt, to taste

2 ounces (55 g) Swiss cheese, shredded

One 5.2-ounce (150 g) package garlic and herb Boursin cheese

4 ounces (112 g) sliced ham

**For the topping**

2 ounces (55 g) pork rinds, crushed

½ cup (50 g) grated Parmesan cheese

Preheat the oven to 375°F (190°C). Grease a 9 x 5-inch (23 x 13-cm) loaf pan with butter to prevent sticking.

In a bowl, season the ground chicken with salt and mix well.

Spread half of the seasoned chicken in the bottom of the prepared pan, pressing it down evenly. Sprinkle the Swiss cheese over the chicken layer. Spread the Boursin cheese evenly over the Swiss cheese layer. Arrange the sliced ham on top of the Boursin cheese.

Cover the filling with the remaining half of the seasoned chicken, sealing the edges to enclose the filling.

Bake the loaf for 25 to 30 minutes, or until the chicken is cooked through and the top is golden brown.

In a separate bowl, combine the crushed pork rinds and grated Parmesan cheese to make the topping.

After the initial baking time, sprinkle the topping mixture over the top of the loaf and return it to the oven for an additional 5 minutes, or until the topping is crispy and golden.

Remove the loaf from the oven and allow it to cool slightly to set.

Slice the loaf into 6 portions.

— DINNER —

# CHEESY CHICKEN CASSEROLE

SERVES 2 TO 4

Butter, unsalted
1 pound (454 g) chicken breasts
Salt, to taste
1 cup (240 g) sour cream
½ cup (116 g) cream cheese
1 ½ cups (180 g) shredded cheddar cheese, divided

Preheat the oven to 375°F (190°C).

Grease a 9 × 9-inch (32 × 32 cm) oven-safe baking dish with butter.

Place the chicken breasts in the prepared baking dish and season them generously with salt.

Bake the chicken in the preheated oven for 30 to 45 minutes, or until the internal temperature reaches 165°F (73°C) and the juices run clear when poked. Cooking time may vary depending on the thickness of the chicken breasts.

While the chicken is baking, in a large mixing bowl, combine the sour cream, softened cream cheese, and 1 cup (120 g) of the cheddar cheese. Mix until smooth and creamy.

Once the chicken is fully cooked, remove it from the oven and let it cool for a few minutes.

Cut the chicken into 1-inch (2.5 cm) cubes and then add the cubes to the large mixing bowl containing the sour cream mixture. Stir until the chicken is evenly coated.

Transfer the chicken and cheese mixture to the prepared baking dish, spreading it out into an even layer.

Sprinkle the remaining ½ cup (60 g) of cheddar cheese over the top of the mixture.

Bake in the preheated oven for 30 minutes, or until the cheese is golden brown and bubbly.

Once baked, remove the casserole from the oven and let it cool for 5 minutes before serving.

— DINNER —

# CHILI

SERVES 2 TO 4

1 pound (454 g) beef (such as chuck steak), cubed into ½-inch (1 cm) pieces

Salt, to taste

3 bacon rashers, cut into small pieces

1 pound (454 g) ground beef

2 cups (480 ml) water or beef broth

**Optional**

1 tablespoon (15 ml) apple cider vinegar

1 tablespoon (16 g) tomato paste

1 tablespoon (7.5 g) chili powder

1 tablespoon (9 g) garlic powder

1 tablespoon (6.9 g) onion powder

2 bay leaves

Shredded cheese, for serving

Sour cream, for serving

Place the beef cubes on a plate and salt them liberally.

In a large pot over medium heat, fry the bacon until it is crispy.

Remove the bacon from the pot, but keep the bacon fat in the pan. Set aside the crispy bacon bits.

Increase the heat to medium-high and add the cubed beef to the pot. Brown the beef, flipping it as needed until it is seared on all sides. Remove the seared beef from the pot and set aside, keeping any fat in the pot.

Add the ground beef to the pot and season with salt to taste. Cook the ground beef until it is browned, then add the seared beef cubes back to the pot. Reduce the heat to low.

Season the beef according to your taste, then pour the water or broth into the pot and bring the mixture to a simmer. Cover the pan with a lid and cook until most of the moisture has evaporated, about 4 hours.

Serve the chili with the reserved crispy bacon bits on top. Optionally, garnish with shredded cheese or sour cream.

— DINNER —

# PARMESAN PORK CHOP BITES

SERVES 2 TO 4

4 boneless pork chops, cut into bite-sized pieces

Salt, to taste

2 tablespoons (28 g) unsalted butter, melted

½ cup (50 g) grated Parmesan cheese

3 cloves garlic, minced (optional)

Preheat the oven to 375°F (190°C) and line a baking sheet with parchment paper.

Season the bite-sized pork chop pieces with salt, to taste.

In a medium mixing bowl, combine the butter, Parmesan cheese, and minced garlic (if using) and stir until well combined.

Using a fork, dip each piece of pork into the Parmesan mixture, coating evenly on all sides.

Place the coated pork bites onto the prepared baking sheet, leaving a little space between each piece to ensure even cooking.

Bake the pork chop bites in the preheated oven for 20 to 25 minutes, or until they are golden brown and cooked through, with an internal temperature of 145°F (63°C).

Once cooked, remove the pork chop bites from the oven and let them cool for a few minutes before serving as an appetizer or main dish.

# COOKED GROUND BEEF PATTIES WITH CHEESE

### SERVES 1 TO 2

1 pound (454 g) ground beef
Salt, to taste
4 slices of your favorite
    cheese (such as cheddar,
    Swiss, or Colby Jack)
Butter, unsalted, for frying

Place the ground beef in a medium mixing bowl and add the amount of salt desired. Mix until well combined.

Divide the ground beef into 4 equal portions. Roll each portion into a ball, then flatten it into a patty shape, about ¼- to ½-inch (6 mm to 1 cm) thick.

Heat a large skillet over medium-high heat. Add a small amount of butter to the pan.

Once the butter is melted, place the patties in the pan and cook for 3 to 4 minutes. Work in batches if needed.

Flip each patty and cook for another 3 to 4 minutes. During the last minute of cooking, place a slice of cheese on top of each patty. Cover the skillet with a lid or aluminum foil to help melt the cheese and cook for 1 minute more, until the patties are browned and cooked to your desired level of doneness.

Serve with toppings or sides of your choice.

— DINNER —

# ROASTED CHICKEN THIGHS

SERVES 1 TO 2

1 pound (454 g) small to
    medium-sized chicken
    thighs
Salt, to taste

Preheat the oven to 400°F (204°C).

Place the chicken thighs in a single layer in an a 9 x 13-inch (23 x 33-cm) baking dish and season generously with salt.

Bake the chicken thighs for 30 to 40 minutes, or until a meat thermometer inserted into the center of the thigh reads 165°F (73°C) and the juices run clear.

Once cooked, turn the broiler to low and crack open the oven door, broiling the chicken thighs for 5 to 7 minutes. Turn the pan halfway through for even browning. Watch the thighs carefully starting at the 5-minute mark to prevent burning.

Remove the chicken thighs from the oven and serve immediately. Optionally, pour the juices from the pan into the bottom of the serving dish to retain all the delicious, fatty flavor.

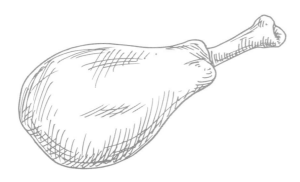

— DINNER —

# ROASTED PORK RIBS

SERVES 1 TO 2

**1 to 2 pounds (454 to 908 g) pork country ribs**
**Salt, to taste**

Preheat the oven to 300°F (148°C).

Place the pork country ribs in a 9 x 13-inch (23 x 33-cm) baking dish and season generously with salt. Cover the baking pan tightly with aluminum foil.

Bake the ribs in the preheated oven for 2 hours.

After 2 hours, carefully remove the pan from the oven and uncover it. Drain any accumulated juices from the pan.

Reduce the oven temperature to 275°F (135°C). Return the uncovered pan of ribs to the oven.

Continue baking the ribs for 30 minutes, then use tongs to flip the ribs and return the pan to the oven for an additional 30 minutes.

Once the ribs are fully cooked and tender, remove them from the oven and serve.

# NO-CARB VANILLA ICE CREAM

### SERVES 4 TO 6

½ cup (120 ml) milk
¼ cup (60 ml) heavy
   whipping cream
1 vanilla bean (optional)
1 egg yolk

In a saucepan over medium heat, combine the milk and heavy whipping cream. If using, slice open the vanilla bean and add it to the pan with the milk mixture. Heat until the mixture begins to simmer.

While the milk is heating, beat the egg yolk in a separate large heat-safe container.

Once the milk is simmering, remove the vanilla bean from the saucepan.

Scrape the vanilla bean seeds into a small bowl and set aside. Discard the outer shell.

While whisking continuously, slowly pour about half of the hot cream mixture to the beaten egg yolk. Pour the egg mixture back into the saucepan with the remaining hot cream mixture, stirring constantly.

Strain the mixture through a sieve into a freezer-safe container. Stir in the vanilla bean seeds.

Continue with either the churning or non-churning instructions below.

**CHURNING INSTRUCTIONS**
Chill the mixture in the refrigerator for at least 4 hours, preferably overnight, to allow it to fully cool and infuse with vanilla flavor.

Place the chilled mixture in the freezer for 30 minutes to slightly firm up.

In an ice cream maker, churn the mixture according to the manufacturer's instructions until it reaches a soft-serve consistency.

Transfer the churned ice cream to a freezer-safe container and freeze for at least 1 hour before serving.

**NON-CHURNING INSTRUCTIONS**
Place the mixture into the freezer for at least 4 hours then serve.

— DESSERT —

# NO-CARB GREEK FROZEN YOGURT

SERVES 4 TO 6

1 ½ cups (360 ml) heavy whipping cream
2 egg yolks
1 ½ tablespoons (23 ml) vanilla extract (optional)
2 cups (460 g) full-fat plain Greek yogurt
Pinch of salt

Place the heavy whipping cream, egg yolks, and 1 tablespoon (15 ml) of vanilla extract, if using, in a saucepan. Over medium heat, bring the mixture to a simmer, stirring occasionally.

In a medium heat-proof mixing bowl, combine the additional ½ tablespoon (8 ml) of vanilla extract with the yogurt.

Remove the egg mixture from the heat and add a pinch of salt. Allow to cool slightly.

Place a heat-proof sieve over the heat-proof mixing bowl and gradually pour the egg mixture through, removing any cooked egg bits. Mix the egg mixture into the yogurt until well combined.

Transfer the mixture to an airtight container and freeze for at least 4 hours or until firm.

— DESSERT —

# CARNIVORE CAKE

SERVES 8 TO 12

**For the cake**
Butter, unsalted
4 (8-ounce/226 g) blocks
  of cream cheese
1 pound (454 g) sour cream
1 tablespoon (15 ml) vanilla
  extract (optional)
4 eggs

**For the topping**
3¾ cups (887 ml) heavy
  whipping cream
Pinch cream of tartar
1 tablespoon (15 ml)
  vanilla extract

**For the cake**
Place all of the ingredients on a countertop in order to come to room temperature.

Preheat the oven to 325°F (162°C).

Prepare four 6-inch (15 cm) cake pans by buttering them well and lining the bottoms with parchment paper.

In a large mixing bowl, use an electric hand mixer to whip the cream cheese on high speed for about 3 minutes or until smooth and creamy.

Add the sour cream and vanilla extract (if using) and mix until well combined.

Add the eggs, one at a time, beating on low speed or mixing by hand, until just combined. Be careful not to overmix.

Pour the cake batter evenly into the prepared cake pans.

Bake the cakes in the preheated oven for about 1 hour, or until the centers are set. Remove the cakes from the oven and allow to cool completely.

While the cakes are cooling, whip the heavy cream with a pinch of cream of tartar and 1 tablespoon (15 ml) of vanilla extract until stiff peaks form.

Once cooled completely, carefully release the cakes from the cake pans and place on individual cake boards or serving plates.

To the top of each cake, add a generous layer of whipped cream.

Transfer the cakes to the refrigerator and chill for at least 30 minutes before serving.

— DESSERT —

# BROWN BUTTER FUDGE

## SERVES 16

*This Brown Butter Fudge is great to use while cooking to add a rich, nutty flavor to your dishes. Or you can also have it on its own as a tasty, buttery snack! I suggest making individual pieces, so you'll need molds or containers for this recipe. You can use silicone molds, ice cube trays, or small ramekins, depending on the shape and size you prefer. If you don't have molds, you can use a larger baking pan or other container and cut the fudge into pieces once it sets. Be careful when removing the set butter from the molds. If using silicone molds, you can simply push the butter out from the bottom. For other types of molds, you may need to run a knife around the edges to loosen the butter.*

**1 cup (2 sticks) unsalted butter**

Cut the unsalted butter into cubes or slices to ensure even melting.

In a saucepan or skillet, melt the butter over medium heat.

Cook, stirring occasionally, until it turns a golden brown color and develops a nutty aroma, about 5 to 8 minutes. Keep a close eye on it to prevent burning.

Once the butter has turned brown and smells fragrant, remove the saucepan or skillet from the heat and allow to cool for a few minutes. Do not let it solidify completely.

Carefully pour the brown butter into your desired molds or containers. Tap the molds gently on the counter to remove any air bubbles and ensure that the butter settles evenly.

Place the molds in the refrigerator and allow the brown butter to solidify completely, about 1 to 2 hours.

Once the brown butter has solidified, carefully remove it from the molds and store in an airtight container in the refrigerator for up to several weeks, or in the freezer for longer-term storage.

— DESSERT —

# PERSONAL NO-CARB CHEESECAKE

SERVES 1

Butter, unsalted
½ cup (115 g) cream cheese
1 teaspoon sour cream
1 tablespoon (15 ml)
    half-and-half
½ teaspoon vanilla extract
    (optional)
1 small egg

Place all of the ingredients on a countertop in order to come to room temperature.

Preheat the oven to 300°F (148°C).

Grease a 4-inch (10 cm) ramekin with butter.

In a small mixing bowl, combine the cream cheese, sour cream, half-and-half, and vanilla extract, if using, until smooth.

Beat in the egg until just combined. Be careful not to overmix.

Pour the mixture into the greased ramekin, smoothing the top with a spatula. Tap the ramekin against the counter to remove any air bubbles.

Place the filled ramekin in a larger baking dish. Fill the outside dish with hot water until it reaches halfway up the sides of the ramekin. This creates a water bath, which helps ensure gentle and even cooking.

Place the water bath and ramekin within it in the preheated oven and bake for 35 to 40 minutes or until set. The cheesecake should be firm around the edges but still slightly jiggly in the center.

Remove the ramekin from the water bath and allow the cheesecake to cool at room temperature for 15 minutes.

Transfer the cheesecake to the refrigerator and chill for at least 2 hours, or until completely firm.

Served chilled.

— DRINKS —

# FATTY COFFEE

SERVES 1

*Fatty coffee is a great way to add more fat to your diet. Especially if you are targeting ketogenic macros, starting your day with fatty coffee can add extra fat at the start of the day to boost your macro ratio. Fatty coffee is also satiating without spiking blood sugar—a great option for those using intermittent fasting strategies.*

**2 to 4 tablespoons (28 to 55 g) unsalted butter, ghee, heavy cream, or 1 egg yolk**
**1 cup (240 ml) freshly brewed hot coffee**
**Dash of cinnamon (optional)**
**Dash of vanilla extract (optional)**

Add your chosen fat to a blender and pour in the freshly brewed hot coffee.

Blend on high speed for 20 to 30 seconds, or until the mixture is frothy and well combined.

Pour the fatty coffee into a mug and enjoy immediately, with a dash of cinnamon or vanilla extract for extra flavor, if you desire.

**Alternative method**
If you do not have a blender, you can use a stick milk frothing whisk to whiz together the fat and coffee in your mug.

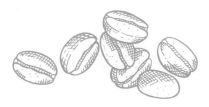

— DRINKS —

# PROTEIN SHAKE

SERVES 1 TO 2

*This recipe involves freezing, so plan ahead!*

1 scoop hydrolyzed whey protein isolate

2 cups (480 ml) milk, divided

3 tablespoons (45 ml) heavy whipping cream

In a blender, combine the hydrolyzed whey protein isolate with 1 cup (240 ml) of milk. Blend until smooth.

Pour the mixture into an ice cube tray and freeze overnight.

Once the cubes are frozen, remove them from the tray and add them to the blender along with the remaining 1 cup (240 ml) of milk and the heavy whipping cream.

Blend the mixture until creamy and well combined.

Pour the creamy shake into glasses and serve immediately.

— DRINKS —

# ELECTROLYTE DRINK

### SERVES 1

*Electrolyte drink mixes are readily available at grocery stores and online retailers. They come in many different flavors and formulations. If you are interested in mixing your own, you can purchase powder mineral supplements at health food stores or online retailers. Personally, I like to use Redmond Real Salt, a mined sea salt for all the benefits of sea salt without all of the microplastics. The following recipe is my favorite mix.*

½ teaspoon Redmond Real Salt

¼ teaspoon magnesium malate powder

⅛ teaspoon potassium chloride powder

1 cup (240 ml) water

In a large glass, add the salt, magnesium malate powder, and potassium chloride powder.

Add the water and mix with a spoon until well combined.

Add ice, if desired, and enjoy!

## Mineral Water Composition

Mineral water, sparkling or flat, can be an excellent way to incorporate minerals while increasing the variety of beverages you drink. Here are the mineral compositions of popular mineral water brands.

**Evian**
Calcium 80 mg/L
Magnesium 26 mg/L
Potassium 1 mg/L

**San Pellegrino**
Calcium 179 mg/L
Magnesium 52 mg/L
Sodium 33 mg/L

**Perrier**
Calcium 55 mg/L
Magnesium 6.8 mg/L
Sodium 9.5 mg/L

**Fiji Water**
Calcium 18 mg/L
Magnesium 15 mg/L
Potassium 5mg/L

— DRINKS —

# BONE BROTH

SERVES 10

2 to 3 pounds (908 g to 1.4 kg)
   raw bones (beef, chicken,
   or pork bones)
Water
1 to 2 teaspoons salt, or
   to taste

Preheat the oven to 400°F (204°C).

Place the bones on a baking sheet (marrow-side up, if applicable) and roast them for 30 to 45 minutes, or until they are well browned.

Transfer the roasted bones to a large stockpot.

Pour enough water into the pot to cover the bones completely. Make sure not to fill the pot to the brim.

Sprinkle in the salt.

Over high heat, bring the water to a boil.

Once boiling, reduce the heat to low. Cover the pot partially with a lid, leaving a small opening for steam to escape.

Let the broth simmer gently for at least 6 to 8 hours. The longer you cook it, the richer and more nutrient-dense the broth will become. Skim off any foam that rises to the surface while simmering.

Once you're happy with the flavor, remove the pot from the heat. Use a fine mesh strainer or cheesecloth to strain the broth, separating the liquid from the bones and any other solids.

Allow the broth to cool slightly before transferring it to storage containers. You can store the broth in the refrigerator for up to 5 days or freeze it for longer-term storage.

## A Word on Seasonings

Many carnivores find that butter and salt are all they need to be satisfied eating meat. Others find they miss the variety and excitement that seasonings can provide. If you are pursuing carnivore for health reasons, eliminating all seasonings will help you establish a baseline of health. If you are eating this way to overcome food addiction tendencies, adding seasonings may help you feel more satiated and help you stick to the diet. Ultimately, whether you use seasonings is a personal choice.

## EATING ON THE GO

Adhering to a carnivore diet in your own home can be relatively easy, especially if you live alone or the people you live with also eat a carnivore diet. Outside of the home can be trickier, but not impossible. Many carnivores enjoy going out to eat, whether it's for variety, convenience, or to share a meal with friends.

Some restaurants are easier to eat at than others, but there is almost always an option available. It should be noted that when eating outside of your home, the food will likely be less ideal than what you could prepare at home—the portions may be smaller, there may be seasonings, and so on. But the imperfect carnivore food you eat is still better than a perfect diet that is impossible for you to stick to.

### Tips for Fast Food Places

Fast food is not an ideal option for carnivores, as this food is typically processed and contains unwanted additives like seed oils and seasonings. However, if occasional fast food makes the carnivore diet more accessible and sustainable for you, choosing to eat fast food when you need to may help you adhere to your nutritional plan.

## To Salt or Not to Salt?

Salt is a major factor in helping you maintain fluid balance. But if you have imbalances in other electrolytes like potassium or magnesium or you don't drink a lot of water, you may find that you do not crave it. While you should eat the way that makes you feel your best, no salt should not be a priority. There is no prize for eating bland food!

Some community favorites include Redmond Real Salt, which is a sea salt free of microplastics as it is mined in Utah. Another favorite is Maldon flaky sea salt, a finishing salt used to add the final, textured crunch to cooked meats. Smoked salt is another incredible way to boost the flavor of any meat dish.

At first glance, you might assume that fast food places are more difficult to order options for your new way of eating. However, because most fast food places have a mix-and-match menu of the same few foods, they often have more flexibility for accommodation and customization. Fast food places are also generally more cost-effective than restaurants, especially if you are doing a lot to customize your order. Here are some tips.

1. **Focus on Meat Options:** Look for items on the menu that already have a meat base. This could include burgers without the bun, grilled chicken, bacon, sausage, shredded pork, or shaved beef.

2. **Skip the Sauces and Condiments:** Many sauces and condiments contain sugars, additives, and other non-carnivore-friendly ingredients. Ask for your order without the sauce, or hand back the condiments given to you at the counter.

3. **Customize Your Order:** One huge benefit to eating at a fast food place is that most allow you to customize your order. Don't hesitate to ask for modifications like removing buns, sauces, or toppings that don't align with your new nutrition plan.

4. **Add Extra Protein:** If you're concerned about getting a large enough portion size, consider adding extra meat to your order. For example, you could order double patties, extra grilled chicken, or add-ons like bacon or an egg.

5. **Don't Order Sides:** Most fast food places offer carb-heavy sides like fries and onion rings. Some offer options like side salads. Generally, fast food sides aren't compatible with a carnivore nutrition plan. Save yourself the hassle and the cost by not making your order a "meal deal."

6. **Be Creative and Flexible:** Fast food menus may not cater specifically to carnivore diets, but you can be creative to meet your dietary requirements. Don't be afraid to mix and match menu items, ask for substitutions, or include add-ons to your order to create a satisfying carnivore-friendly meal.

Ultimately, fast food options can add variety and convenience to your 30-day carnivore boot camp, but they may not be strict carnivore, and customized orders can add up quickly. To be successful at carnivore, eat the meat you like, can afford, and makes you feel your best. Try to eat most of your meals at home, but when you do dine out, make the best choices available to you.

### Tips for Restaurants

As a carnivore, eating at a restaurant can be similar to dining at a fast food place, but it sometimes requires a little more nuance. However, with a little mindfulness and communication, it is totally doable! Here are some tips to help you navigate the menu and enjoy your dining experience.

1. **Look at the Menu Ahead of Time:** Many restaurants have their menu available online. Review the menu before you go to see what meat-based options they have available. Be sure to look at the sides and appetizers too!

2. **Talk to Your Server:** If you are comfortable with telling your server about your dietary preferences, you can tell them before you order. You can ask if they are able to make certain substitutions or have other ways to accommodate your preferences. Asking, "What is the best way to get a big plate of meat?" may also help them generate a creative solution for you.

3. **Focus on Meat-Centric Dishes:** Look for entrees that feature meat as the main component. This could include steak, grilled chicken, seafood, eggs, or pork. It goes without saying that you should avoid dishes that are heavily based on carbohydrates or other plant-based ingredients.

4. **Ask for Substitutions:** If needed, you can ask for modifications to menu items to better suit your new way of eating. This might include omitting starches or vegetables from a dish, requesting sauces on the side, and asking for extra meat.

5. **Consider Appetizers or Sides:** Many appetizer and side options at restaurants are carb-based, but there are often meat-based options as well.

Charcuterie boards, bacon-wrapped scallops, shrimp cocktail, chicharrons, and sides of bacon, sausage, or eggs are all options. You can order these as intended to start or complement your meal, or you can order them as your meal.

6. **Enjoy Yourself:** Dining out is not just about the food—it's also about the experience. Focus on enjoying the company you are with, the ambience of the restaurant, and the opportunity to try new meat dishes.

By planning ahead, communicating your needs, and being creative, you can enjoy a restaurant meal as much as you did before you transitioned to a carnivore diet. Most people choose to pursue a nutritionally dense diet so that they can live their best possible life. Even when dining out, you can choose to support your health and your lifestyle by adhering to your 30-day carnivore boot camp.

## Carnivore Travel Tips

Travel can make carnivore more logistically difficult. So, making a plan and knowing your options ahead of time can be vital to your success. Ideally, you'll be able to bring foods to have on hand that meet your new nutritional preferences, but in a pinch, here are some carnivore-friendly travel tips.

Good choices include whisps (baked cheese snacks), jerky, beef sticks, cheese sticks, pork rinds, eggs, whole milk/keto protein shakes, and fully cooked bacon/sausages. Others include prepped meat (burgers, bacon meatballs, meat muffins), wraps, hard-boiled eggs, canned or pouch chicken, tuna, salmon, or sardines, dehydrated meat, and lunch/deli meats. Always check the ingredient list on premade products. One reason carnivore is so beneficial is that it removes processed foods from your diet, so don't unwittingly bring them back in.

### Flying Domestically and Internationally While Carnivore

While you can find food options at an airport, like burgers at a dining place or beef jerky at a convenience shop, it can be very expensive. Instead, pack food ahead of time, if possible, or partake in an extended fast. If non-carnivore food is offered on the flight, decline it, as it is much easier to resist temptation when it isn't sitting right in front of you.

At first glance, flying internationally may seem impossible as a carnivore. However, bringing carnivore options onto an international flight is just as easy as a domestic one. If you bring prepared meat with you, make sure you eat it before going through customs. Depending on the country you are traveling to, you may not be able to bring meat with you.

## TRANSITIONING TO 30-DAY CARNIVORE: THE ROLE OF FASTING

Now that you've learned about what to eat, what to shop for, and when to eat, let's talk about taking a break from eating, specifically daily intermittent fasting and long-term

fasting, typically for 24 hours. Whether you are pursuing a carnivore way of eating for fat loss, improved energy, or other health benefits, you may be well served by incorporating fasting into your new diet strategy.

### Benefits of Fasting

Fasting has been researched for a long time; ancient Greeks used it to manage seizure disorders, and recent research continues to provide evidence for the benefits of fasting, including weight loss, autophagy, and inflammation control.

#### *Weight Loss*

There are a few different ways in which fasting can help contribute to weight loss. Generally, fasting limits calorie consumption because you are restricting eating times. It can be difficult to eat as many calories as you usually would in a shortened time frame.

Fasting can also induce a ketogenic state, where your body switches to using fat for fuel and oxidizes body fat for energy. Fasting can also improve your insulin sensitivity. By reducing the number of insulin spikes you have from eating, you allow your body to recover from the insulin spike fully before eating again.

It should be noted that excessive fasting can work against your weight loss goals. Your body needs protein and fat to generate energy. If your diet is so restricted in calorie consumption or consistent food intake that it runs out of dietary protein and fat, your body may start catabolizing, or breaking down, your muscle tissue. While many people want to leverage carnivore for potential fat loss benefits, it is important to feed your body enough so you don't lose muscle mass.

### Autophagy

Autophagy is a natural bodily process that breaks down and recycles damaged or dysfunctional cells. This process is essential to maintain health and homeostasis because it removes misfolded proteins, damaged mitochondria, and intracellular pathogens. Autophagy also regulates various processes, including cellular remodeling, adaptation to stress, and energy metabolism regulation. Dysregulation of the autophagic process is associated with neurodegenerative disorders like Alzheimer's and Parkinson's, cancer, metabolic disorders, and infectious diseases.

Fasting supports autophagic function by stimulating autophagy as a survival mechanism. It promotes the breakdown and recycling of damaged cellular components. During intermittent or extended fasting, the body switches from glucose to fat as an energy source, breaking down fat cells and triggering autophagy. Research suggests that intermittent and prolonged fasting support autophagy, potentially offering health benefits such as improved cellular repair.[69] However, prolonged fasting and calorie restriction can lead to muscle catabolism, a secondary autophagic process that breaks down healthy cells for energy.

### Inflammation Control

Another benefit of fasting is inflammation reduction and management. Fasting decreases production of pro-inflammatory molecules such as cytokines. It can also promote the production of anti-inflammatory molecules and enhance cellular resilience to stress. As we've seen, fasting also stimulates autophagy, removing old, dead cells and intracellular pathogens.[70] Old, dying cells can release free radicals, further contributing to inflammation.

For people experiencing chronic illness, chronic inflammation can play a role in many of the symptoms they experience. For example, symptoms of arthritic conditions that cause inflammation of joints, tendons, and ligaments can be managed with intermittent or extended fasting.[71] It should be noted, however, that managing symptoms is not necessarily treating the root cause of the disease, and should be considered a band-aid, not a cure.

## Types of Fasting

The two types of fasting are intermittent and extended. Both forms come with benefits and one may feel more aligned with your lifestyle than the other. You can always try both to see which one feels most supportive of your goals. That said, fasting is not a requirement of a successful carnivore diet, and if it feels difficult and hard to adhere to, you may find that fasting is not supportive of your new way of eating.

### Intermittent Fasting

Intermittent, or daily time-restricted, fasting is a very accessible form of fasting. It is very popular in the carnivore community, possibly because many people adopt this way of eating through paleo or keto, where intermittent fasting is also popular. Intermittent fasting requires a shortened eating window. Rather than eating throughout the day, you decide on a typically 4- to 6-hour window in which you will eat all your meals. This provides an 18- to 20-hour fasting time period that provides many of the weight loss, autophagy, and inflammation control benefits previously discussed.

While most people participate in the shorter 4-to 6-hour eating window, you can start with a longer, 8- to 10-hour eating window and still reap some benefits. Over time, you may choose to further reduce your eating window. Ultimately, the only way to find the eating window that works best for you is to try it!

Incorporating intermittent fasting should be a lifestyle (not a nutrition) choice at the beginning of your carnivore journey. For example, your work or activity schedule may naturally require it. Once you have fully transitioned to a carnivore diet, you can consider the benefits of incorporating intermittent fasting to support your goals.

### Extended Fasting

Typically, extended fasting is considered any fast lasting more than 24 hours. Some people promote extended fasting as a way to reduce inflammation or manage binge-eating disorders. However, fasting for these purposes may treat the symptoms but does not address the root cause of the issue, whether it is discovering the cause and resolving inflammatory triggers or addressing disordered eating behaviors.

Extended fasting is not ideal for people transitioning to a carnivore diet. While there is some evidence that extended fasting can promote weight loss, it isn't productive for long-term improvements in body composition. Extended fasting increases cortisol, the stress hormone. It can also promote muscle wasting as the body consumes muscle for energy.

The longer the fast, the greater the risks. Fasts lasting longer than 24 hours should be supervised by an appropriate medical provider. For the purposes of your 30-day carnivore challenge, an extended fast should be considered a 24-hour fast performed no more than once a week.

To prepare for an extended fast, make sure you are well-fed and well-hydrated. During your fast, consider supplementing electrolytes to overcome lightheadedness caused by electrolyte imbalance. If at any point your fast causes any undesired symptoms like fatigue, irritability, headaches, or any other feeling you don't want to experience, you can stop your fast and eat a nourishing meal of meat!

## BIOHACKING

Another way to enhance the benefits of your 30-day carnivore boot camp is biohacking. Biohacking is the practice of changing your lifestyle and environment to optimize your performance. This practice can take many different forms, including dietary approaches, exercise modalities, regulating your limbic system, modifying your daily routine, improving your sleep hygiene, and managing stress. While some practices are well researched, others are experimental and should be approached with caution.

## FASTING
## Longer Isn't Better

When it comes to fasting, longer isn't necessarily better. The longer you fast, the greater the risk of unwanted side effects. Side effects like muscle degradation from calorie restriction, electrolyte imbalance from dehydration, and overeating as a response to excessive hunger can become amplified by longer fasting periods.

## Metabolic Stress

Appropriate metabolic stress from activities like weight-lifting and high-intensity cardio like sprinting are beneficial if your goals are to improve performance, build muscle, and build metabolic resilience. With these forms of exercise, a scaled approach and proper form are especially essential. If it is your first time practicing these sports, hire an appropriate fitness professional or coach to guide you through best practices for your chosen exercise.

### Dietary Biohacking

A carnivore diet could easily be considered a form of dietary biohacking. By only eating the most nutritionally dense food group you are optimizing your dietary approach. Incorporating other strategies, like electrolyte supplementation and intermittent fasting, are other examples of dietary biohacking.

### Fitness Biohacking

Biohacking your fitness routine typically involves balancing metabolic stress (see sidebar) with practices that support the regulation of your limbic system (see following). Most people pursuing a fitness regimen are typically doing so with a specific goal in mind—for example, fat loss, muscle building, increased flexibility, or improved endurance. Understanding what you hope to achieve through a fitness regimen may help you decide which exercise modality is best for you, your lifestyle, and your goals.

Gentle exercise, which can include activities like walking, yoga, tai chi, and leisurely bike riding, are also supportive of many fitness goals. Especially if you want to gain flexibility and mobility or achieve better hormone regulation, focusing on gentle movement can be the most efficient way to achieve those results. If you are just beginning to pursue fitness activities, prioritizing gentle movement, and gradually building endurance and mobility, will allow you to begin incorporating more high-impact movements.

## Limbic System Biohacking

The limbic system is a network of brain structures that help regulate emotion. Limbic system activation, or the fight-or-flight response, happens during times of stress as a way to prioritize survival. A fight response can lead to symptoms like hypotension, feelings of anxiety, reduced digestive motility, and difficulty concentrating. Symptoms of a flight response include many of the fight response symptoms but can also include avoidance and a tendency toward isolation.

This activation of the limbic system and response is healthy in small doses. After all, our bodies and minds adapt to high-stress and risky environments so that they are best prepared to fight or flee as the situation requires. For people who have experienced trauma or chronic unwellness, their limbic system is activated a disproportionate amount of time and they become stuck in this fight-or-flight response. Unfortunately, the physical and psychological stress of maintaining a hypervigilant state can lead to chronic inflammation, anxiety, and mental dysregulation.

The antidote to limbic system activation is parasympathetic nervous system activation. The parasympathetic nervous system is responsible for promoting recovery and rest. It slows heart rate, lowers blood pressure, increases digestive rate, and improves mental clarity as a way to maintain homeostasis in the body. For those who are trying to achieve healing or improve fitness performance, intentionally entering a parasympathetic state accelerates recovery, helping you achieve your goals.

Brain retraining is the process of performing daily practices that help rewire neural pathways to switch your default from fight-or-flight to parasympathetic regulation. There are formal brain retraining programs that can be purchased online. However, finding a practice that resonates with you, in a way that you could see yourself incorporating daily, will be the most effective one for you. Mediation, gratitude journaling, learning a new language or instrument, breathwork, and gentle exercise are all forms of limbic retraining that can be easily incorporated into most lifestyles.

Limbic practices take just that—practice—for them to be effective. Focus on one small, accessible, daily practices that you can adhere to. Over time, as you build the habit of limbic practices, you can add layers of other limbic practices to further strengthen your parasympathetic system response.

## Lifestyle Biohacking

One of the most accessible formats of biohacking is making small lifestyle changes that you can incorporate daily. In the biohacking community and discourse, the focus is often on extremes—extreme acquisition of products, extreme time commitments, or putting your body through extreme stressors—to achieve results. This style of biohacking has its place, but for the average person, a more sustainable approach can still help them achieve results. These practices, such as taking Epsom salt baths and getting more sunlight, can take minimal time, money, and energy but improve your overall quality of life.

**Calming the Nervous System with Epsom Salt Baths:** Those familiar with biohacking may be familiar with the cold-plunge craze. Cold plunges have many touted health benefits, such as improved exercise recovery, alertness, and immune function. By plunging your body into cold water for a period of time, you are forcing your body to rapidly adapt to an extreme environment, which can translate to more resilient metabolic function.

If you have experienced trauma or chronic illness, you can reap more benefits through a more parasympathetically supportive biohacking practice. Warm Epsom salt baths are relaxing and supportive of metabolic function. Warm baths can stimulate the parasympathetic nervous system, which will optimize rest and recovery.

When added to warm bathwater, mineral-rich Epsom salt can promote muscle relaxation, wound healing, sinus relief, improved sleep, and skin hydration.[72] Epsom salt baths are a relaxing and accessible biohacking practice that you can easily incorporate into your weekly routine.

**Getting More Sunlight:** There are many benefits to sunlight exposure. Exposure to sunrise and sunset, or low-horizon sunlight, stimulates alpha-MSH, a hormone that performs many functions in the body and can support healthy sleep, sex hormone function, fat loss, and immune function.[73] Sunlight during the day, under the correct UV conditions, stimulates vitamin D synthesis from cholesterol. Vitamin D is a precursor to many hormone functions in the body and chronically low vitamin D levels is often associated with poor health outcomes.[74] Exposing your skin to sunlight for 15 to 30 minutes per day can help promote healthy vitamin D production.[75]

Tracking your sun exposure with an app that accounts for your skin type and propensity to tan can help you reap the benefits of sun exposure without risking sunburn. D Minder is one such app and can help estimate vitamin D levels by also tracking vitamin D supplementation.

### Sleep Hygiene Biohacking

Sleep is one of the easiest things for modern people to deprioritize. Sleeping less seems like an easy strategy to gain back more hours in the day. A good night's rest is wildly underrated. And a consistent, prioritized sleep schedule can be one of the most powerful tools you can use to take your performance to the next level.

Sleep hygiene is creating a routine that puts you in the best possible position for a good night's rest. Figuring out your optimal sleep routine will take some trial and error, but here are some suggestions to get you started.

**Consistent Sleep and Wake Times:** Falling asleep and waking up at the same time every day is one of the best ways to establish consistent sleep quality. Also, having the same routines before bed and upon waking will give you a baseline for what a good night's rest feels like for you. If you have a poor night's sleep and there were no variations to your routine, you will know to check other possible causes for disturbed sleep, such as nutrition or caffeine intake.

**Cold and Dark:** Some studies have shown that sleeping in a cold, dark room can help improve sleep quality.[76] Typically, it is suggested that the optimal temperature for sleeping is between 60° and 67°F (15.5° and 19.5°C). Use blackout curtains or a sleeping mask to eliminate light.

**Avoid Blue Light at Night:** Light comes in many different colors. Blue light is associated with the color of daytime and the big blue sky. Our lizard brain associates blue light with wakefulness, and daytime exposure to blue light can help regulate our wake-sleep cycles. However, in our modern society, we are also exposed to blue light from electronic screens, such as televisions, computers, and phones.

Blue light exposure at nighttime can dysregulate your wake-sleep cycle. Turning off electronics a couple of hours before bed, or wearing blue-light-blocking glasses in the evening, can help promote optimal sleep.

## Stress Management Biohacking

There are entire industries devoted to stress management. Chronic stress is like living in a house in the TV show *Hoarders: Buried Alive*, with clutter surrounding you at every turn, filling up your life, and causing you to stumble and fall.

Stress management is like going into a hoarder's home with $1 million worth of organizational supplies from The Container Store and neatly tidying your clutter away. The clutter is still there, filling your home and your headspace, but it is just better organized and tucked away into little compartments.

The more effective approach to stress might be digging in, finding the source of the stress, and eliminating it from your life. Sometimes this isn't possible—you can get rid of debt or relocate to a better apartment, but you can't necessarily get rid of your kids, your spouse, or your job.

What you can control is your thoughts. Your thoughts control your feelings and your feelings control your actions. So, to a certain extent, we can choose not to react negatively to stressors by using stress management techniques to help us survive until the clutter can be cleared away. Here are some ways you can clear the clutter in your mind.

**Mindset Management:** Acknowledging and addressing your thoughts and emotions is a process called mindset management. Instead of ignoring or resisting stress, greet it, welcome it inside, come to an understanding, and walk it out the door. Although this process might sound counterintuitive, in practice it helps you decide and control your reactions to stressors. One practice I like to use is reframing, or changing the way I feel about a situation by choosing better thoughts to support the way I want to feel. Here's how to do it. I suggest using a journal, but you don't have to.

1. How am I feeling right now? (one word)

2. What thought is making me feel this way?

3. How do I want to feel? (one word)

4. What thought do I need to have to feel this way?

Let me show you how this works. For many starting the carnivore diet, they have a history of chronic dieting. So, their reframing practice might look something like this:

1. Right now I am feeling: overwhelmed

2. The thought that is making me feel this way is: I will never lose this excess body fat

3. I want to feel: successful

4. The thought I need to have to feel this way is: I am a person who is investing my energy into learning and following a carnivore diet that will work for my health history, my journey, and my goals!

Reframing might seem like an easy way out. But personally, I have never felt better during stressful times by beating myself up about it more. A good friend once told me to speak to myself as though I were a small child. You wouldn't berate a small child for trying their best, so don't talk to yourself that way either!

Learning to process your emotions and manage your mindset are powerful tools that can help you succeed in many areas of your life.

**Remove the Unnecessary:** In addition to the big scary obvious stressors filling our days, everything we consume is another potential piece of clutter we are adding to our lives. Be selective in what you consume: what you buy, what you watch, whom you speak to, what you read. Everything you allow into your life is either helping you or harming you. You get to choose what you allow in, so choose wisely. Here are some things you can do to eliminate unnecessary clutter in your life.

- Unsubscribe from unwanted emails.

- Unfollow or mute social media accounts that make you feel less-than.

- De-clutter your junk drawer.

- Remove old and unworn clothes from your wardrobe.

- Clear out unneeded files from your desktop.

Decluttering your life doesn't have to be one massive action; it can be the accumulation of one tiny task you complete every day.

## CHEAT SHEET
## Stress Hacks

At the end of the day, there will still be stressors that absolutely cannot be avoided. Here are some hacks that can help you get through them a little bit easier.

**Morning Workouts:** Working out in the morning has been shown to temporarily spike cortisol levels but then reduce your overall cortisol baseline for the rest of the day. By working out in the morning, not only do you produce less stress hormone throughout the day, but you also get to start your day with a win.

**Posture:** Our posture is biofeedback to our brains about how we should feel. If we are hunched over and look defeated, our brain thinks we should feel defeated. Sit up straight, take up space, hold your head high, and let your brain think you are a badass, because, well, you are!

**Humor:** Anytime you feel like the stress is all too much, turn on your favorite comedic TV show. Especially if you have already seen every episode multiple times, laughing floods your brain with happy hormones, and who doesn't want more of those?

Many people, our ancestors included, have been able to achieve incredible health without the use of gadgets to optimize their wellness. Anyone promoting biohacking techniques with a discount code to the product they are selling shouldn't be your only source of information regarding that particular biohack. Instead, do some research to see whether you feel incorporating the biohack will truly make a large enough improvement to your overall health to justify the investment. Much like a carnivore diet, there is no *one* perfect biohacking routine—there is just the perfect biohacking routine for you.

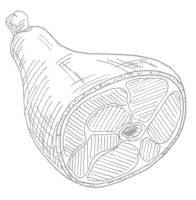

# 4

# OVERCOMING OBSTACLES TO YOUR SUCCESS ON A CARNIVORE DIET

As you begin your 30-day carnivore boot camp, you'll find that, just like in the rest of life, you'll encounter obstacles. However, this doesn't mean that you should use them as an excuse to avoid making positive changes in your life. Instead, use obstacles as an opportunity to prove to yourself that you are tenacious and resilient and that you can do difficult things, persevere, and get positive results. In this chapter, we'll take a look at the most common obstacles to a successful carnivore diet and the tools and resources to overcome them.

## TRANSITIONING TO CARNIVORE AND MEETING NUTRITIONAL NEEDS

Carnivore is a nutritionally whole diet, meaning it contains all the nutrients you need to survive and thrive. However, as you embark on your carnivore journey, you might get feedback and concern from friends, family, and coworkers about what you're eating. At this point, you'll want to remember that the carnivore diet provides all the macro and micronutrients you need to live and maybe even educate them about this too.

### Am I Getting Enough Vitamin C?

After four years of eating a carnivore diet, nothing shows me how conscious I have become of nutrition misinformation as when people ask about my diet. When it comes to vitamin C, the question usually goes like this: "Won't you get scurvy without vitamins from fruit?" It's a fair question. We all were taught that sailors were once at risk of scurvy without sufficient vitamin C intake from fresh fruits.

Scurvy is a medical condition caused by lack of vitamin C. Early signs of vitamin C deficiency include a lack of energy, followed by painful swelling and flexion, poor wound healing, gum disease, and, without correction, death. Scurvy is not common in most first-world nations, but is one of the hallmark diseases caused by malnutrition seen in underdeveloped countries to this day.

To answer this questions, it's first important to understand that vitamin C and glucose compete for pathways in the human body. The Recommended Daily Allowance (RDA) for many vitamins is based on diets that include glucose, but we likely need much less dietary vitamin C in its absence. Additionally, fresh meat (not just liver) contains enough vitamin C to satisfy daily requirements for many people following a carnivore diet.

If you are concerned about your vitamin C intake and/or would like to set the minds of your loved ones at ease regarding your possible scurvy, supplement with vitamin C. However, be sure to obtain vitamin C supplements from a reputable source that uses ascorbic acid, as commercially produced citric acid is often manufactured from black mold, a known human toxin.[78]

### Sailors, Scurvy, and Vitamin C

There is evidence that sailors knew fresh meat had enough vitamin C content to help them prevent and even recover from scurvy.[77] Despite tragic symptoms of painful, swollen, discolored legs, a 1902 expedition to the Arctic was able to reverse signs of scurvy within two weeks after gaining access to fresh seal meat.

Native cultures, like the Inuit, who hardly ever, if ever, eat plant foods, also do not display signs of scurvy. Anthropological researcher Vilhjalmur Stefansson and author of *Not by Bread Alone* studied traditional Inuit culture and their diet for decades and didn't find any cases of scurvy.

### Other Helpful Minerals to Ease the Transition

**Magnesium** is necessary for muscle contractions and nerve functioning, and can reduce anxiety, improve digestion, balance fluid levels, and support quality sleep. If you notice muscle cramping or tingling in your fingers and toes, you may want to consider supplementing with magnesium. If you are taking magnesium citrate and experiencing loose stools, try a different form of magnesium like magnesium malate, chloride, or glycinate.

**Potassium** helps maintain fluid homeostasis, keeping blood pressure levels stable. It also aids muscle function and is especially useful in regulating heart contractions. If you are experiencing constipation, muscle fatigue, or heart palpitations you may want to consider supplementing with potassium. Chicken and clams are high in potassium, or consider adding an electrolyte supplement that contains potassium.

## Reduced Mineral Content in Soil = Need to Supplement with Carnivore

While one of the common arguments for a carnivore diet is that it is nutritionally complete, most carnivore experts and thought leaders recommend the supplementation of minerals. That's because the reduced mineral content in meat is caused by the reduced mineral content in soil.

Ancestrally, when most modern plant agricultural fields were forests and plains, there was a diverse ecosystem that remineralized soil through the circle of life. A variety of animals and plants would die in those environments and become the diverse nutrient-rich soil that new plants would grow from that new animals could eat.

Modern, non-regenerative agricultural practices strip soil of its nutrients by planting singular crops that cannot remineralize soil effectively.[79] Since our plants contain fewer minerals, the animals that eat them contain fewer minerals too, which ultimately means all humans, regardless of their diet, will likely need to supplement electrolytes (see page 117).

*Note:* If you are experiencing any heart symptoms, immediately contact your health care provider.

**Sodium** also helps maintain fluid homeostasis in the body and is essential for muscle contractions and nerve signaling. Sodium is depleted by cortisol, so you may notice you crave more salt when you are stressed. Sodium may also play a role in uric acid levels; while not dangerous in the absence of carbs, it is important to drink water to thirst to maintain appropriate fluid balance in the body.

If you are experiencing fatigue, muscle weakness, or restlessness, you may want to consider supplementing with sodium. I choose refined mined salts like Redmond Real Salt because sea salt often contains toxins and microplastics from human garbage and waste being pumped into the ocean.

## NEW CARNIVORE CONCERNS

Some people starting a carnivore diet may have concerns about getting tired of eating meat, eating too much meat, or craving carbs. While eating a variety of meats prepared in a variety of ways can easily help you overcome these concerns, there are some strategies you can use to make the transition to a carnivore diet even easier for yourself.

## Meat Aversion

Transitioning to a carnivore diet can lead to unfamiliar appetite issues. Some people experience a ravenous hunger for meat as they begin to eat nutrient-dense foods for every meal. Others may experience meat aversion, meaning they cannot stomach the thought of eating meat for every meal even though they are hungry. Meat aversion, if experienced, is typically temporary.

If you choose a meat-based, or more relaxed, approach to a carnivore diet, using seasonings or seed oil–free condiments like hot sauce or mustard may help get you through this transition period. Ideally, and especially if you are leveraging a carnivore diet to understand your health baseline, you'll want to eliminate all plant toxins from your diet.

However, the carnivore diet you can stick to because it is appetizing to you is more effective than giving up because it feels too difficult. Leverage spices and condiments as needed at the start. Later on, you can always choose to eliminate plants as flavorings.

New carnivores can also use cheese, sour cream, Greek yogurt, and other dairy to entice the appetite. Cheese adds calories as well as flavor to almost any meal. Cheese also triggers dopamine receptors and can be a helpful replacement for previous go-to carb-filled snacks when cravings strike.

As you start a carnivore diet, don't limit yourself to the meat you think is nutritionally best if it isn't appetizing to you. Many people consider grass-fed and finished beef the nutritional gold standard, and in the carnivore community, people can feel pressured to avoid processed meats like sausage and non-ruminant animals like chicken, pork, or fish. In previous chapters, you learned about the benefits of eating a variety of meats instead of hyperfixating on finding the most nutritionally dense meat. All animal protein contains essential vitamins and nutrients and eating a variety of meats will provide a variety of flavors and textures. The imperfect meat you eat will be more effective at helping you transition to a carnivore way of eating than the perfect meat you have no appetite for. As I say, eat the meat you crave, when you crave it.

## Eating Too Much: Over-Satiation

If you find that eating a carnivore diet makes you full too quickly, it may be helpful to review the macronutrient ratios you are consuming. Protein is much more satiating than fat. Because protein is 4 calories per gram compared to fat's 9 calories per gram, you need to eat a lot of protein in weight to equal the same amount of fat. This makes protein voluminous, meaning it is literally filling.

An easy way to ensure you are eating enough is to eat fat first so that you don't fill up on protein before you consume all the calories you need. Eating fat first is often easy—for example, you can eating an egg's yolk before you eat the white of a fried or hard-boiled egg. If you are eating a food that is mixed fat and protein, like scrambled eggs, adding fat in the form of butter or other animal fat can be an effective way to up the calories without making you feel overly full.

## When to See Your Health Care Practitioner

The greatest use for the carnivore diet is to discover your nutritional baseline in the absence of dietary toxins from plants and processed foods. If you cannot overcome meat aversion issues, you may want to investigate underlying health issues such as bile production or gastrointestinal issues. Work with the appropriate health care practitioner to resolve any remaining health issues you experience after establishing a new health baseline on a carnivore diet.

## Carb Cravings

Carb cravings or addiction, a perceived dependence on carbs for satiety, can derail your 30-day carnivore boot camp if it goes unchecked. Know that if you experience an intense craving for carbs, your body may be adjusting to its new energy source or it could be old mental patterns coming into play.

As you transition to using fat for fuel by eliminating carbohydrates, your body may crave the old, easy energy source at the start. As your body adapts to a new energy source, do your best to ignore the cravings. Typically, giving in to them often leads to bingeing. Instead, keep your favorite carnivore foods at the ready. For me, that was bacon prepared and in the fridge, ready to crush any cravings with a satiating salty, fatty bite. Over time, you will notice these cravings die down, and as you enter ketosis, you will experience more stable, consistent energy.

Carb cravings also occur as part of a habit or an emotional response. Habitual carb cravings are the ones that occur when you relate a part of your routine with carbs. For example, you used to watch TV and eat popcorn every night. The easiest way to overcome habitual carb cravings is to change your routine. Instead of watching TV, read a book or build a puzzle. Simply removing the activity that you associated with carbs may be all you need to stay on track.

Emotional cravings are when you reach for food to soothe emotional discomfort. Instead of stuffing your emotions down with food, try addressing emotional distress with productive responses, like therapy, meditation, or journaling. Old mental

## Artificial Sweeteners

Artificial sweeteners can help some people overcome sugar cravings, while others find them to be a trigger to eat actual sugar. Over time, the goal should be to eliminate all artificial sweeteners to establish a true health baseline.

## Cheese to Curb Cravings

Cheese and dairy are often controversial when it comes to the carnivore diet. While cheese is an animal product, it is processed and can contain a small amount of carbs, so for people who are using carnivore to uncover a health baseline, eliminating cheese can be supportive of their health goals.

However, the proteins in cheese work along the same pathways in the brain to create a dopamine response similar to the one with sugar. Therefore, cheese can be a helpful "hack" to overcome carb cravings during the transition period. It is controversial because many carnivores believe we should avoid all processed foods, even if they are from an animal source. Only you will know whether eating cheese feels correct for your health history and your goals.

patterns will be relearned over time as you experience the benefits you are looking for through this way of eating.

## DEALING WITH THE KETO FLU

During your transition from a standard American diet to a 30-day carnivore boot camp, you might face flulike symptoms as your body adjusts from relying on carbohydrates for energy to utilizing fat. Those familiar with the ketogenic diet may have heard of the keto flu.

For most people living in the modern Western world, the normal way of eating has become a diet of mostly carbohydrates. Carbohydrates turn to glucose in the body, and glucose is a cheap and easy energy source. While carbs are great for immediate energy needs, they are less efficient at long-term energy requirements. Any glucose not immediately utilized is stored in the liver as well as shuttled away to fat cells for storage. If an energy deficit occurs, the body can convert the stored glucose back into energy.

There are a couple of downsides to using carbohydrates for energy. For one, because energy supply spikes immediately after eating carbs and then excess is stored away, it is hard to achieve a feeling of consistent energy and vitality. If you don't meet the energy requirements needed to utilize the stored glucose, you can experience fat gain and even fatty liver disease (see page 29).[80]

Diets that reduce carb intake, like keto and carnivore diets, force the body to use other energy sources: protein and fat. Carbohydrates are the only nonessential dietary macronutrient. Since protein can be converted to glucose in the liver through a process called gluconeogenesis, your body can meet its glucose requirements.

Fats are able to be leveraged for energy through a different metabolic pathway that produces ketones. Ketones are a much more stable and consistent energy source because they don't rise and fall dramatically the way glucose does.

Keto flu is not experienced by everyone and there are steps you can take to mitigate the effects should you experience any adaptation symptoms. Electrolyte supplementation, intermittent fasting, and eating enough protein and fat can all ease any keto flu symptoms you experience as you transition to a carnivore diet.

### Electrolyte Supplementation

Electrolytes are minerals in your body that carry electrical charges. They're carefully balanced to maintain homeostasis between the interior and exterior of your cells. Electrolyte imbalance can cause symptoms such as fatigue, lethargy, excessive thirst, frequent urination, dry skin, headaches, dizziness, weakness, constipation, and nausea. New carnivores often find that supplementing with electrolytes such as magnesium, potassium, and sodium can be helpful. That's because going carnivore means you're eating a lot less sugar or glucose and this affects your electrolyte balance. In a carb-centric diet, excess glucose is stored in cells to be used for later energy requirements (or turned into body fat if that energy is never required). Glucose is hydrophilic, meaning it loves to hold on to water.

If you are transitioning to a carnivore diet from any other way of eating, you are going from a state of eating some carbs to eating negligible carbs. As you continue to consume only protein and fat, your body will start to release the excess glucose stored in your cells. Along with the glucose, you will release the excess water it is holding on to. This explains the "whoosh," or rapid weight loss experienced by many people at the start of their new low- or no-carb diet. Along with the water, you lose those essential minerals necessary to keep your body in hydration homeostasis. The sudden change in hydration balance can lead to electrolyte imbalance.

Over time, you may find that you need less supplementation as your body adapts to your new way of eating. It's always best to follow the advice of your health care practitioner when it comes to mineral supplementation. Too little can make you feel lethargic while too much can stop your heart.

Electrolyte imbalance is easy to treat with an electrolyte supplement, commonly comprised of sodium, potassium, and magnesium. There are products on the market that make electrolyte supplementation easy, but you can also make your own for a fraction of the price. I use ½ teaspoon of fine mined salt (I like Redmond Real Salt), 400 mg of powdered potassium chloride, and ¼ teaspoon of powdered magnesium malate mixed into at least 8 ounces (240 ml) of water no more than three times a day.

I take a biofeedback approach to electrolyte supplementation. Meaning, I take supplements when I crave them. This approach is especially effective if you supplement with unflavored electrolytes because craving the supplement is indicative of your body craving the minerals, rather than craving an artificial flavoring or taste.

Before deep-diving into the world of nutrition, I thought electrolytes meant salt. Since then, I have learned that while salting to taste is a great strategy for me to maintain my electrolyte balance, it isn't as effective as supplementing potassium and magnesium in addition to sodium.

## Intermittent Fasting

One way that you can overcome keto flu symptoms more quickly is by intermittent fasting and eating enough protein and fat to support your body's transition from using carbs for energy to using fat for energy. This is called "ketosis," or a metabolic state produced by leveraging fat for energy. Once you are in ketosis, you will experience the benefits of fat as an energy source. If you are eating enough fat while limiting dietary carbs, you will achieve ketosis.

One easy way to enter a ketogenic state more quickly is by intermittent fasting. Intermittent fasting is the practice of restricting caloric intake to a shorter time frame within the day. Strictly speaking, everyone intermittent fasts overnight. While you are sleeping, you are not eating. Eating breakfast is typically how we break our overnight fasts. Intermittent fasting encourages shorter eating windows like 6 to 8 hours. An example of an intermittent eating schedule could be only consuming foods between 11 a.m. and 7 p.m. or 8 a.m. to 3 p.m. (See page 153 for more on intermittent fasting.)

Intermittent fasting has many reported benefits.[81] Most notably for our purposes, intermittent fasting helps people enter a state of ketosis more quickly. As your body utilizes all available glucose in your

### Ketosis, Not Ketoacidosis

While they may sound similar, ketosis and ketoacidosis have nothing in common. Ketosis is the metabolic state of using fat for energy instead of carbohydrates. Ketoacidosis is a life-threatening condition most commonly experienced by people with type 1 diabetes. This condition develops when you have an insulin deficiency.

bloodstream, it transitions to using ketones for fuel. Limiting the frequency of glucose presence in your bloodstream by limiting your eating windows can expedite the transition to primarily using ketones as fuel.

## Eating Enough Protein and Fat

While your body is transitioning to using fat as your primary energy source, your body still needs adequate protein to function optimally. You may not need carbs in your diet, but your organs do need glucose converted from protein in a process called gluconeogenesis. You must eat enough protein if you are leveraging gluconeogenesis to convert protein to glucose. Your brain needs glucose; it cannot run only on ketones. If you do not consume enough dietary protein to meet your brain's glucose requirements, your body will harvest protein from the only source it has available: your muscles.

While many people eat a ketogenic diet to lose weight and may be tempted to reduce calories to expedite weight loss, they are hamstringing their progress by catabolizing their hamstrings. Avoid muscle loss by using a calorie calculator[82] to determine an appropriate amount of calories for you and your goals.

Make sure you're also eating enough easy-to-access dietary fat as you transition away from carbs. As I've said, your body will convert the glucose it needs from protein, and the remaining protein will break down into amino acids, essential building blocks for the human body. The majority of protein you consume will be used for amino acids, not energy. Your body's main source of energy, therefore, will be fat.

Eating enough fat is always important, but especially as you are starting the diet and dealing with symptoms of keto flu. Supplementing animal fats like butter, tallow, lard, chicken fat, or fatty cheeses can help boost the fat content of your meals. Similarly, choosing fatty cuts of meat, like rib-eye, 80/20 ground beef, chicken thighs, fatty pork chops, and fatty cold-water fish can help ensure you are eating enough dietary fat to mitigate the symptoms of keto flu.

## DIGESTIVE CHANGES AND CHALLENGES

Gastrointestinal health is vital to our overall well-being.[83] In recent decades, researchers have discovered the gut-brain axis, or the connection between gastrointestinal system and mental health. Research shows that over 50 percent of our dopamine,[84] the "feel good" chemical in our brain, is created in our gastrointestinal tract. Gastrointestinal issues are also commonly found in people experiencing autoimmune disease.[85] For people with chronic gut-health issues, carnivore can be a powerful tool that eliminates gut-irritating plant toxins.

Carnivore can help you better understand your gut health baseline. By eliminating excess inflammation caused by glucose and removing excess plant toxins as a confounding factor to your GI health, you can better understand which symptoms need to be addressed through interventions outside of nutrition. Leveraging carnivore as a tool to better understand the health issues you are experiencing can help you more efficiently pursue and achieve root-cause healing.

For others, carnivore can completely heal underlying gut issues like candida or SIBO. By eliminating the glucose and carbohydrates these bacteria feed on, you can reduce or eliminate bacterial overgrowth in your body. The Harvard Carnivore Study of anecdotal stories from carnivores had many reported instances of gut healing,[86] with gut issues being the second-most common reason after autoimmune diseases for people to pursue eating a carnivore diet.

Often, an unexpected benefit to the carnivore diet is less frequent bowel movements. Since our food is so nutritionally efficient, and without the unnecessary volume of indigestible high-fiber carbohydrates, we're able to digest and eliminate much more efficiently. This isn't an obstacle,

## Digestive Enzymes and Bile Acid Production

Digestive enzymes like ox bile can help regulate your bile acid production. Bile acid is created in the gallbladder and is essential to your body's ability to digest fat. For those transitioning to a lower-carb diet, it may take their body time to adapt to higher bile acid requirements for the higher dietary fat contents of their diet.

Low bile acid can cause nausea or fatigue after eating, as your body is trying to digest food without the help of bile acid breaking down the fat molecules. Another sign that you are not producing enough bile is clay-colored bowel movements, which can indicate a low-level of bile in your intestines.

necessarily, just a point to be aware of. You do not need to be concerned as long as you are having a bowel movement every day.

Having said that, often when people switch to a low-carb diet they experience gastrointestinal changes. Some find they're more constipated than they used to be. Others find their stools are looser than they used to be. Regardless of the changes you are experiencing with your bowel movements, there are strategies you can practice to normalize them again.

An important thing to note is that after onboarding onto a carnivore diet, your bowel movements should normalize on their own. If, after 30 days of eating a carnivore diet, you are still not experiencing improvements in your bowel movements, you have uncovered a health baseline that exhibits an unregulated gastrointestinal system. At this point, you will want to work with an appropriate health care practitioner to identify your GI issues and guide you through a protocol to heal them.

### Constipation

As previously mentioned, a benefit to the carnivore diet is less frequent bowel movements. Constipation is the inability to pass stool; if you are not uncomfortable or in pain, then you may just be experiencing this unique benefit of the diet. One bowel movement per day seems most typical for people following a carnivore diet.

For those experiencing constipation, there are a couple of options to help you go. Eating rendered fat can help increase motility in your digestive system. Melt butter, tallow, or other animal fat onto your food just before eating. Another option is to increase your salt and magnesium intake. Hydration and electrolyte balance are important factors that positively impact gut motility. Electrolyte supplementation may be all you need to move things along (see page 117).

If you are experiencing pain or discomfort from your constipation and the recommendations above do not help you have a successful bowel movement, you may need to seek medical intervention. Speak to an appropriate health care practitioner for guidance on resolving uncomfortable or consistent constipation issues.

### Loose Stools

Loose stools are the most common issue experienced by people transitioning to a carnivore diet. The sudden elimination of fiber is the number one reason most people experience loose stools. That's because your body needs to adapt to the sudden lack of roughage it typically has to process through your GI tract.

Another reason for loose stools is due to the adjustment of your gut biome. Our gut biomes are incredibly complex, diverse, and rapidly adjusting in response to dietary changes.[87] While our understanding of the gut biome is currently limited, we do know that it is incredibly responsive and begins adapting to dietary changes in as little as 24 hours.

If you are experiencing loose stools, eliminate all liquefied fat (try cold butter, suet, or other animal fat instead). Cold fat is digested more slowly and will slow down motility in your digestive tract. Allowing your food to cool enough so that the fat begins to solidify before eating may also help prevent sudden, urgent loose stools.

Beverage timing also affects digestive health. If you drink a beverage with your meal, you are effectively increasing your GI motility through hydration. Separate beverages from mealtimes by at least an hour to reduce gut motility and loose stool issues, especially as you transition into the diet. Over time, you may find that you can become more lax in your beverage timings as your body better adapts to your new way of eating.

If you experience persistent or painful loose stools after transitioning to a carnivore diet, you have uncovered a new health baseline that reveals possible GI issues. Seek the advice of an appropriate health care practitioner to help you diagnose and treat the root cause of your GI distress.

## STRATEGIES FOR STICKING WITH CARNIVORE

The greatest obstacle to any challenge is our own mind. Henry Ford said, "Whether you think you can or can't—you're right." Your mindset can be your #1 fan or your worst enemy. To set yourself up for success, know the obstacles you might encounter and plan how you will deal with them. This proactive mindset can be the difference between success and failure on a carnivore diet.

You can do hard things. Just look at the lifetime of hard things you have accomplished so far! You can do this 30-day challenge for yourself, and when you do, you will have even more evidence that you can do hard things and choose yourself and your goals over momentary pleasure. Let's explore some of the strategies for sticking with carnivore so that you can be successful with this new way of eating. Remember, you're worth the effort it will take to get used to taking care of yourself.

## Understanding Changes in Sleep Patterns

Some people experience changes in their sleeping patterns as they transition to a carnivore diet. Your body is adapting, so this is to be expected. The good news is that over time many carnivores report that they have better sleep than they did pre-carnivore. Some of the causes of changes in sleep patterns are blood sugar spikes, "meat sweats," and biphasic sleep patterns.

### Blood Sugar Spikes

As your blood sugar begins to regulate, you may experience midnight wake-ups. This may be due to blood sugar spikes. Eating some cheese, which is high in casein protein and digests slowly, can help prevent blood sugar spikes and may help you stay asleep through the night.

### Meat Sweats

Have you ever heard of meat sweats? Protein takes a lot of energy to digest, so eating a high-protein meal before bed may result in waking up sweaty and hot in the middle of the night. Avoid eating large amounts of protein before bed to avoid the meat sweat phenomenon.

### Biphasic Sleep

Throughout history people often woke up in the middle of the night, visited with family and friends for a couple of hours, and went back to bed.[88] But today, waking up in the middle of the night is considered a sleep disorder and is usually medicated. For some people following a carnivore diet, biphasic sleep may be a normal sleep pattern; the important thing is the total amount of quality sleep, not necessarily how consecutive it is.

### Use Systems, Not Goals

At the end of this challenge, when you have designed the perfect carnivore diet for you, your next step is to make it as easy as possible for yourself. As popularized by the book *Atomic Habits* by James Clear, setting systems to complete the actions that move you toward your goals is a great way to achieve success. For example, if your goal is to avoid eating out, you could create a system to meal prep twice a week so that you always have food on hand. You know what they say: When you fail to plan, you plan to fail.

## Make Better Choices

Perfectionists seem to have a common trait of feeling like if they cannot do something perfectly, they would rather not do it at all. Making small, positive movements will always get you further toward your goals than never moving at all.

Instead, focus on doing the best that you can in any situation. Meal prep when you can, and when you can't, use the dining out guide in chapter 3 to select the best options available to you at a restaurant or on the go. Buy your preferred protein/fat ground beef, and when you can't, add supplementary fat or drain excess fat to get to the ratio you prefer. Your journey doesn't have to be perfect; all you have to do is keep moving forward.

## Review Your Goals and Accomplishments

As I've said, you're a person who can do hard things. You are a person who chooses to take care of yourself. You are a person who moves toward your goals. You know how I know this? Because something led you here. You have lived with enough health concerns or excess body fat to bring you here, and those are hard things to live with. You decided to invest in this challenge for your health and your future, and that is an amazing gift to give yourself. You got this far! Just reading this book is an amazing and important step in the direction of your dreams.

Keep building on the momentum you have started. Every time you experience a win or a new carnivore benefit, take note!

Every time you add another item to the list of benefits you have experienced through your new way of eating, review all of your accomplishments so far.

## Educate Yourself

You are actively working on this one! Learning about the carnivore diet can be an overwhelming experience and there are many rabbit holes to go down. This book is intended to help you get started in the way of eating that will support you and your goals best. Over time, as you learn more and possibly uncover health issues through your new health baseline, you can tweak your diet and pursue different carnivore-adjacent approaches to achieving your best health.

All of this is to say, there is a lot of content out there. Not all of it will serve you and your journey. Stick to the basics and critically assess any variations to see whether they make sense for you before diving into the newest trends.

## Find Community

Having a community to lean on that understands the experience you are going through can make a huge difference to the success of your journey. Even if you are introverted, make an effort to connect with one or two people in the community. Make them your accountability buddy to share all or your highs and lows with. Knowing you have someone to support you and whom you can offer support to in return will further help you connect to your new lifestyle. A carnivore community will also help you as you encounter questions or skepticism from well-meaning friends and family, the topic of the next section.

## HOW TO DEAL WITH QUESTIONS ABOUT GOING CARNIVORE

As you embark on your 30-day carnivore journey, you may need to talk about your reasons for adopting this new way of eating to others at home, at work, and in social situations.

On the one hand, you want to avoid preaching about a diet that appears extreme to others. On the other hand, you may become tired of people asking you how you poop without fiber. Even if you avoid telling people about carnivore for your own peace, once people near you start to see your transformation, the results will speak for themselves.

Still, there will be people and situations in your life where you cannot avoid talking about your new way of eating. Especially when it comes to loved ones, this can be a sensitive topic. Many people believe that meat is bad and plants are good. They may be concerned for your well-being and your health. Judgment of the carnivore diet comes from a good place for most people, whether it is concern for you, for animals, or for the planet.

Understanding that the person you are speaking to believes they are right and has your best interest at heart can help reframe and retemper the conversation. It can be helpful to approach the conversation with the thought "I used to think this way too."

Going into what might be a difficult conversation with that level of empathy helps you stand your ground while appreciating the views of the other person. In our society, we are inundated with information and it can be difficult to discern what is true, or more importantly, true for you.

### Share Your "Why"

One strategy for talking with loved ones is to explain your "why" for pursuing a carnivore diet. Remember your why? (See page 24.) Sharing your why is a powerful tool that will allow them to empathize with the choices you are making for yourself. Next, provide some basic evidence as to how this way of eating supports your why.

The people closest to you will better understand the health, fitness, and wellness struggles you have had in the past. Many people are familiar with not feeling as fit as they would like to and it is easy for them to empathize with this goal. Understanding why this way of eating is important to your success in overcoming those struggles will help garner their support. Framing your new diet to loved ones in this way can give them better context for your new way of eating: You are using your diet as an adjunct therapy to your healing.

Still, some people may view carnivore as an extreme way to achieve your goals. Let them know that you are exploring carnivore for 30 days to see what it can do for you, and that you are open to pivoting if you do not begin to see results. This will assure them that you are not dogmatic in your approach.

Our society is becoming more aware and accepting of mental health struggles. For those pursuing carnivore for the mental health benefits, you may consider explaining to loved ones the mental health battle you are fighting. We can only give to others what we have of ourselves. Improving our mental well-being allows us to give better versions of ourselves to others and our loved ones deserve the best version of us we can give to them.

At the end of the day, your reasons for pursuing carnivore are your own—for your own health, fitness, and well-being. While it is always good to listen to the feedback or concerns from people you love and respect, it is also good to choose yourself. And as previously said, the results speak louder than words.

### Do Your Homework and Share What You've Learned

Another strategy for dealing with loved ones who question your new way of eating is to do your research ahead of time. What convinced you to try this diet in the first place? By no means should you have to defend the way you choose to eat, but it can be helpful to educate your loved ones about why you think this way of eating is the right choice for you. Having a couple of data points or references ready to go when you are asked questions about the diet shows your loved ones that you are approaching this new way of eating thoughtfully.

There is much more information and awareness regarding low-carb and ketogenic diets these days. Explaining that

## Carnivore and Criticism

To many, carnivore will seem like a nontraditional diet. Some people might be skeptical of your new nutritional approach. Starting a new way of eating is a big life change, and the scrutiny of others will not make that transition feel any easier. If possible, avoid conversations about diet and nutrition, especially with people you think will be critical of your new way of eating.

carnivore is a simplified variation of a low-carb diet that will allow you to reap the benefits without complicated meal planning and tracking may be a great starting point. Since people already have some context for this way of eating, it can help reframe carnivore from a restrictive extreme to a simplified known.

The Harvard Carnivore Study[89] is another excellent piece of evidence to share with loved ones. The study is anecdotal, but there are over 2,000 participants reporting similar stories of healing and wellness success through this way of eating. The participants were required to have been following a carnivore diet for six months or more, far longer than your own 30-day challenge.

When a loved one asks you a question about your new way of eating that you don't feel confident answering, tell them ,"I

## Talking About Carnivore with Acquaintances

In many ways, speaking to acquaintances about your new dietary strategy is much easier than communicating with loved ones. With loved ones, typically more context is needed and more concerns need to be addressed. With acquaintances, you can choose the depth of conversation and the amount of context you wish to provide to them.

When talking to acquaintances about your new way of eating, you can keep the conversation as surface level as you want to. "I am doing an elimination protocol" and "I am trying to determine the source of some possible food allergies" are both great phrases to use.

Alternatively, you may come to a point where you experience so much healing and growth from a carnivore way of eating that you want to share it with others. If people ask curious questions and you feel comfortable sharing more, give them some insight into your new way of eating. Avoid berating their own way of eating or going on tangents about the corruption of the food system, as these tactics can make people feel defensive and assume you are a crazy conspiracy theorist.

don't know, but I will find out." You won't always have all the answers, but acknowledging your ignorance and openness to learning more may help your family and friends understand that you are not taking an inflexible approach to your new way of eating. You are an excellent example to them of staying open and adapting to new information.

### Instead of Carnivore, Try Telling Them It's an Elimination Diet

People are becoming more and more aware of food allergies and sensitivities. In the past few decades, we have seen the rise of gluten-free, low-FODMAP, and anti-inflammatory diets. It is very common for people to expect their food sensitivities (and even preferences) to be accommodated.

If you must talk to someone about your new way of eating and you don't want to have an in-depth conversation about it, tell them you are doing an elimination protocol. Elimination diets are commonly used to help identify food sensitivity issues by stripping the diet back to a bare minimum and then adding back foods one at a time to gauge reactions. Carnivore is, by definition, an elimination protocol because it eliminates seed oils, grains, plants, and, if you choose, dairy.

Not only is this an accurate representation of carnivore, but it also inherently implies that you do not plan to eat so narrowly forever. And again, if after 30 days you choose to continue a mostly carnivore lifestyle, you can then speak to the results you achieved through a carnivore way of eating.

### Choose Yourself

Ultimately, there may be people in your life who will not support your new dietary approach. And that is okay. I am sure your loved ones sometimes make decisions you don't understand either. You know why you are pursuing carnivore, and you know what outcomes you hope to achieve with your nutritional choices. If those outcomes make you a better person, everyone in your life, including your loved ones, benefit from it.

So stand your ground. At the end of the day, you are a free agent. While you may appreciate the wisdom of others, you are the one who has to live with the decisions you make. The conversation about your diet isn't to convince them to allow you to eat this way; it is to inform them of the choice you have made for yourself.

If your loved ones really push back against your decision, you can always tell them you are just trying it out for 30 days to see what happens. Again, communicating that you are open to alternative approaches may be all they need to hear to quell their concerns. Once the 30 days are over, if you decide to move forward with carnivore for a longer period of time, explain the benefits you experienced over the past 30 days. It is hard to argue with good results.

## NAVIGATING SOCIAL OCCASIONS

Social events are opportunities for bonding and connection, often revolving around shared experiences, including food. People eating a carnivore diet might worry about feeling excluded or left out of these communal experiences if their dietary restrictions prevent them from fully participating in shared meals or culinary experiences.

In chapter 3, you learned about all the options for eating at home, at restaurants, and on the go. One of the biggest psychological hurdles to overcome with a new carnivore way of eating is believing that unless it is perfect, it will not work. The imperfect meat you eat is more effective than the perfect but unobtainable idealized diet you cannot stick with. This is never truer than navigating a carnivore diet while in social situations.

Social situations can be difficult and awkward. But nothing will make you feel worse than your own discomfort. A lot of the conflict you anticipate from social situations is largely in your own mind. Most of the time people aren't looking at you; they are busy worrying that everyone is looking at them.

Wisdom comes with age and also helps you worry less and less about what other people think of you. The people who truly care about you won't care that you insisted on bringing your own food to dinner. They won't care that you order chicken wings at lunch, and they certainly won't care if you bring an amazing meat and cheese platter to their party.

## The Value of a Support System

You may find that no one in your life supports your new way of eating. Feeling alone can make this journey more difficult than it needs to be. Plugging into an online carnivore community and finding a tribe of people who understand and support the decision you have made can be the key to sustainable success on a carnivore diet.

The carnivore community is active in many social spaces. There are formal groups you can pay a membership fee to join. There are free forums on sites like Facebook and Reddit. The Instagram community shares a lot of food inspiration pictures and recipes. Occasionally, there are even carnivore meetups, retreats, or conferences you can attend. There are many different options to connect with other carnivores. Finding a community that you resonate with can be life-changing in and of itself.

While there is a lot of value in being a member of a larger group, many people also find it helpful to connect with a few individuals and create a smaller tribe. Choose people you want to do this journey with, who are supportive of your positive choices, and whom you can lean on when you struggle.

Not only will you feel the value in having a support system, but you will also feel the incredible reward of being someone else's go-to source of support. Somehow, helping other people thrive on their carnivore journey can make your own that much more meaningful. For me, I found community on online carnivore forums on Reddit and eventually started an Instagram page that allowed me to find new carnivore friends.

However, social situations can be more difficult in the sense that you have less control over every detail. But the challenge of being given a situation and making the best choice possible builds your confidence in knowing that you can live your best life anytime, anywhere.

Social occasions do not need to become a stressful obstacle in your 30-day carnivore boot camp. There are many carnivores across the globe navigating social situations every day, and you can too! Using some simple strategies and tools, navigating social situations while on a carnivore diet becomes a piece of steak!

### Social Occasions at a Venue

There are pros and cons to being invited to a social event hosted at a location other than someone's home. It is a cultural norm for us to expect food to be incorporated at most celebrations and events. If you are involved in the planning of an event, you may be able to influence the choice of activity or restaurant.

## Going Carnivore and Social Events

You might think that eating a carnivore diet will add restrictions to your life. Your new nutritional needs require additional navigation, especially in social settings. However, your new dietary preferences do not have to be an obstacle in your social life. Many carnivores find they are still able to attend the events they love, with very little inconvenience to others or themselves.

If possible, suggest an activity that doesn't revolve solely around food. Instead of going to brunch to catch up with friends, suggest a morning hike. Instead of going on a lunch date, suggest a walk through a park or a quick game of mini golf. Instead of hosting a dinner party, invite people over for an early afternoon board game party and prepare a charcuterie snack to share. There are alternatives to food-centered gatherings and they often incorporate more movement and connection than simply sharing a meal together.

For gatherings that require food, if you are helping to plan the event, suggest carnivore-friendly restaurant options. Some types of restaurants provide more carnivore options than others. Steakhouses, Mexican restaurants, and sushi places all have more easily accessible carnivore options (see the restaurant ordering suggestions below).

If you cannot impact the decision, you can still explore the options at the venue by looking online and planning ahead. And, worst case scenario, you can eat beforehand or bring carnivore-approved snacks with you.

**Plan Ahead:** If you are invited to a social event and the location is already set, scope out the menu ahead of time. Most restaurants have their menus available online. Take a peek at the menu and try to find two or three options that will work for you. That way, even if an option is not available the day of the event, you will already have decided upon a backup meal. This will help you go to the event with more confidence—you are choosing your goals without sacrificing social connections to do so!

**Eat Beforehand:** Even when menus have a seemingly carnivore-friendly option available, know that the portion size may be small for the cost. Eating a light meal before going to the event will suppress your hunger enough to feel satiated by a likely smaller portion size. A good pre-event meal will be one that is filling without feeling too heavy. Eating a meal rich in protein with fat will help you feel satiated without feeling overly full. Consider eating a plate of scrambled eggs, chicken thighs, or some fatty cold-water fish like salmon before you eat out.

Worst case scenario, if you end up with a larger portion of meat than you

## New Carnivore and Digestive Symptoms When Eating at Events

Earlier in this chapter we discussed some of the potential digestive issues you may encounter as you transition to a carnivore diet. An additional consideration to attending events may be managing any digestive symptoms you are experiencing. If possible, avoid events during your first week of eating a carnivore diet. Allow your gastrointestinal system to adjust to your new way of eating. If an event cannot be avoided, scope out where the restrooms are when you arrive at the venue to prevent a panicked search should the need suddenly arise.

expected, you can always ask for a take-away container to bring it home with you to enjoy later. This is a much better option than sneaking non-carnivore foods from someone else's plate because you are still hungry.

## Social Occasions at Someone's Home

In some ways, eating at someone's home is easier than dining at a restaurant. If the host is accommodating, ask if you can bring something to share (more about this in a minute); this way, you gain more control over what you are eating.

In other ways, eating at someone's house can be more difficult. You may have to explain your nutritional preferences to people. If you are bringing something to share, you may have to plan and prepare a dish. If you'll be at their house for a long period of time, you may need to bring additional options for yourself. The good news is that there are easy strategies you can use to make this the best possible experience for yourself.

**Don't Get Too Hungry:** The number one tip for staying on track when you go to events is to not let yourself become too hungry. Eat a light meal beforehand, bring snacks or a dish to share, and have an escape plan ready if you start to feel hungry. When you are hungry, you're more likely to sacrifice your goals and reach for not-ideal foods. Curbing hunger can prevent bad decisions.

**Bring Emergency Snacks:** Emergency snacks can help you stick to your new way of eating. Even if you bring food to share, bringing private snacks just in case is a good preventive measure. Precook bacon to keep in your car or purse just in case other meat options run out.

You can excuse yourself as needed to partake of your snack should hunger pangs begin to strike mid-event. Emergency snacks are a great way to prepare for events of unknown length, so that you don't feel forced to make bad diet decisions or have to leave an event early.

# CHEAT SHEET
## Dining Out

Most restaurants (except plant-based venues) have some carnivore options on their menus. They may not be ideal or as clean as the carnivore options you have available to you at home. Dining out should be an occasional necessity for most carnivores, and eating meat, even imperfectly prepared or seasoned meat, is still moving you toward your goals.

If a restaurant's menu doesn't appear to have a ready-to-go option, you may just need to ask for a side of meat or no bun and toppings with your burger. Some of these options are not 100 percent ideal, but they are better than not eating carnivore at all and will allow more flexibility and therefore sustainability in your diet. When in doubt, ask the waiter, "What is the cheapest way for you to bring me a plate full of meat?"

### Fast Food Restaurants
- Plain burger with cheese, no bun
- Breakfast sandwich with egg, bacon, and cheese, no bread
- Grilled chicken nuggets
- Chicken wings (ask about breading and seed oils)
- Sous vide egg bites
- Meats by the pound off a catering/ BBQ menu
- Build-your-own taco bowl with meat, cheese, and sour cream

### American Fare
- Plain burger with cheese, no bun
- Chicken wings (ask about breading and seed oils)
- Meatloaf (ask about what is in it)
- Grilled or baked pork chops
- Grilled or baked chicken

### Mexican Restaurants
- Ask if you can "double your protein" or add protein as a side and order multiple sides of beef, chicken, or pork
- Fajitas (order shrimp and beef for more volume at lower cost)
- Molcajete typically includes meat cooked in a tomato-based broth, so avoid if you are sensitive to the toxins in tomatoes

### Asian Restaurants
- This is a great choice because entrees are often separate from the carb options
- Mongolian beef, no sauce
- Grilled chicken, no sauce

### Sushi Restaurants
- Sashimi (this can become really expensive, so try to go during happy hours or if they have a special)

### Italian Restaurants
- Oysters
- Sausages
- Ask what is in their meatballs
- Order a chicken Caesar salad without the salad
- Scrape the toppings off of meat lover's pizza with no sauce

### Mediterranean Fare
- Side of gyro meat

### Carnivore-Friendly Restaurants
- Barbecue
- Brazilian steakhouse
- American steakhouse
- Chicken wing venues that fry wings in tallow

**Explain Your New Way of Eating:** Using the strategies discussed earlier in this chapter, explain your new way of eating to your host. If they are a close loved one, you can get into the details of why you are pursuing a carnivore diet. If they are an acquaintance that you prefer to not have an in-depth discussion with, you can share as simply as saying, "I am doing an elimination protocol to help identify food sensitivities I have been experiencing." Most people are reasonably understanding of dietary restrictions, and some will be happy to accommodate them.

Once you explain your dietary preferences, offer to accommodate them yourself. Telling your host about your dietary restrictions is a courtesy to let them know that you may not partake in all of the food offered to you. Letting them know that you do not expect them to create an entirely separate and special menu for you is also courteous. Ultimately, your new way of eating is your choice and you are responsible for feeding yourself.

If the host insists on providing an option for you, give them the bottom line of your diet: you only eat meat cooked without seed oils. This will give them the opportunity to assess whether this is something they can or want to accommodate. If they are still happy to prepare an option for you, make suggestions of easy-to-prepare meals or snacks that you commonly make at home. Grilled meat, pan-fried burgers, and slow-cooked roasts all require relatively little preparation and attention.

If a host accepts your offer to let you cook for yourself, tell them what you plan

## Carnivore and Cultural Practices

Some events come with a cultural expectation to eat certain things. Your participation in these cultural practices is totally up to you! Rituals that involve food are not about nutrition, they are about partaking in a cultural or belief system. Taking part in these practices doesn't make you less of a carnivore. The purpose of carnivore is to help you be the healthiest, best version of yourself. It's not to win a medal for being the perfect carnivore at the cost of practicing cultural rituals that are a fundamental part of what makes you who you are.

to bring for yourself and if you will need any supplies or time to prepare it. For example, if you plan to bring precooked meat, tell them you may need to borrow a frying pan for 10 minutes to heat it up. This will allow the host to plan ahead for any resources you will need to successfully feed yourself.

The goal is to remain a courteous guest while adhering to the nutritional plan you have created for yourself. Communicating your needs, setting expectations, and taking responsibility for your own nutritional goals will allow the host to feel they are supporting you while not creating any inconvenience for them.

**Bring Something to Share:** It's nice to bring a dish to share when you're invited to someone else's home. Not only will you be sure to have something you can eat, but you can also share a tasty, nutritious option with others while contributing to the host's menu. Some easy-to-bring dishes you can bring are roasts, meat and cheese casseroles, and charcuterie boards.

Roast meat is a nice option to bring and share. Typically, the preparation is simple: bake, braise, or slow-cook a large cut of meat until it becomes tender. Allow it to cool enough to firm up, then slice and serve! Most roasts taste equally good hot or warm. The pan drippings can be reduced down in a skillet and strained to serve alongside the meat as an *au jus*.

Casseroles are holiday gathering staples for many and can be easily modified to accommodate carnivore requirements. Consider modifying an already beloved meat and cheese-based casserole recipe and eliminate the plant ingredients. If you do not have an easy to adapt casserole recipe on hand, search the internet for "carnivore casserole recipe" or "meat and cheese casserole recipe."

Charcuterie, or a meat and cheese board, is also a nice option to share. Here are some ideas:

- Assorted cured meats like salami, prosciutto, and pepperoni

- Assorted cheeses like Manchego, aged cheddar, Brie, and goat cheese

- Cracker alternatives like cheese baked into crackers, thinly sliced dehydrated meat, or jerky

- You can choose to add or admit other traditional charcuterie accouterments like fruit, jams, olives, peppers, traditional crackers, and mustard

Dessert is a tricky subject on a carnivore diet. If you are including sugar alternatives in your diet, a sugar-free cheesecake is a carnivore-friendly option that you can share. If you're not eating sugar alternatives, but still want to bring a dessert you can eat while others enjoy theirs, bake a cheesecake without sugar or sweetener. If you've been carnivore for a significant period of time, even unsweetened cheesecake can taste like an indulgent treat!

**Prepare a Meal for When You Get Home:** Before heading out to the event, make sure you have prepared carnivore food in the fridge for you to come home to. If you become hungry during the event and have no options available to you, the knowledge of delicious, healthy food at home can prevent you from making impulse decisions that prevent you from reaching your goals.

**Focus on Progress, Not Perfection:** If you are at an event and stray from your new way of eating, all is not lost! You can still pick up where you left off and make better nutritional decisions from that point forward. Remove the pressure of absolute perfection from your diet.

# CHEAT SHEET
## Holiday Gatherings

When you're invited to a social event or holiday party, it may seem impossible to stick to your goals. However, it's totally possible for you to live a normal social life while maintaining boundaries around your health and wellness. Here are some tips to follow.

- **Tip 1** Have a specific goal with a deadline. It is so much easier to stick to your goals when you are specific. If you want to lose weight, decide how much and what day you would like to achieve that by.

- **Tip 2** If you are not the host, inform the host of your dietary restrictions. This will help prevent awkwardness on the day of the gathering.

- **Tip 3** Provide your own dietary options for every stage of the meal. I love any excuse for a magnificent charcuterie board! Also, plan on taking an additional meat side to share.

- **Tip 4** Eat before you go and bring snacks along. Part of the appeal of holidays like Thanksgiving is the overstuffed feeling, and bringing your own snacks just helps it along.

- **Tip 5** If you are making dishes for the meal, don't make your favorites! You can make something delicious for everyone else and it doesn't have to be your favorite thing (looking at you, cheesy potatoes).

- **Tip 6** If you are alone for the holiday, make the best of it and prepare yourself a feast of all your favorite foods that meet your nutritional goals.

- **Tip 7** Make "better alternatives" to traditional fare, such as bacon-wrapped asparagus instead of a green bean casserole. However, it is best to plan to stick to meat.

- **Tip 8** If you do eat something that does not meet your nutrition goals, forgive yourself and keep moving forward. You are not a failure for having a slice of super-delicious pumpkin cheesecake. You are a human, trying to improve your life.

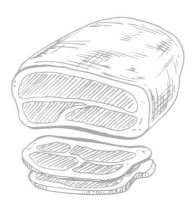

Eating an imperfect, but generally nutritious diet 90 percent of the time will help you reach your goals much faster than the perfect but inaccessible diet you are only able to maintain 10 percent of the time. Eat the best you can at any moment and know that the next time you need to make a choice about what to eat, you are given a new opportunity to choose yourself and your goals.

### Hosting a Carnivore Event

Many carnivores, as they begin to see the benefits of their new nutritional choices, want to share their way of eating with others. One beautiful, inclusive, and noninvasive way of sharing your new diet with others is to host a party or event and serve your new favorite foods. One common objection to a carnivore diet is how difficult people assume it is to navigate in everyday life. Hosting an event with easy, delicious, and accessible carnivore dishes can exemplify how easy carnivore really is.

Your carnivore event doesn't even have to be overtly carnivore. You might be surprised by how easily you can host friends and family without identifying a nutritional theme to the items being served. An easy way to do this is by inviting people over for grilled meats, smoked meats, or a roast. Ask other people to bring side dishes and no one will know that, as the host, all you are serving them is meat.

You don't have to feel like your dietary choices are restricting you from hosting events for the people you love. You can serve people food you can feel good about without feeling as though you are forcing your nutritional beliefs upon them.

Navigating social interactions with your new way of eating requires open communication, preparation, and a willingness to assert your dietary preferences. You can do this while also being respectful of others' choices and hospitality. Planning ahead, bringing carnivore-friendly dishes or snacks, and confidently but kindly explaining your dietary choices can help hosts and other guests feel more comfortable at social events while adhering to your 30-day carnivore boot camp.

## TURN OBSTACLES INTO OPPORTUNITIES WITH A GROWTH MINDSET

When I think of carnivore, I think of resilience. Adopting a carnivore diet helps you develop a more resilient mindset by allowing you to practice overcoming obstacles, like the social challenges of eating a specific diet. Facing challenges from a foundation of health and vitality can help you see all obstacles as opportunities for growth.

A growth mindset is a valuable skill to develop. People with a growth mindset believe that they are a constantly evolving, able to learn, adapt, and become better over time. This mindset allows you to become the best possible version of yourself by overcoming obstacles through your own tenacity and ingenuity. Here are some tips on approaching obstacles with a growth mindset.

1. **Embrace Obstacles:** View challenges as opportunities for growth rather than setbacks. Approach obstacles as a chance to learn and improve.

2. **Focus on Problem Solving:** Instead of dwelling on challenges, direct your energy toward finding solutions. Break down the total obstacle into smaller, manageable tasks and tackle them one step at a time.

3. **Stay Open-Minded:** Be flexible to adapting your plans and strategies when faced with challenges. Staying open-minded allows you to explore different approaches and find creative solutions to overcome obstacles.

4. **Remember Your Why:** Keep things in perspective by reminding yourself of your long-term goals and the bigger picture. Remind yourself of past experiences where you successfully overcame obstacles to build evidence in your ability to overcome current challenges.

5. **Be Gentle with Yourself:** Practice self-compassion during difficult times. Avoid self-criticism and negative self-talk, and instead, be kind to yourself by treating yourself with understanding and acceptance.

6. **Get Help:** Don't hesitate to reach out to friends, family, or mentors for support when facing challenges. Seeking support from others can provide valuable insights, encouragement, and perspective to help you overcome obstacles.

7. **Celebrate Your Wins:** Acknowledge and celebrate your achievements, no matter how small. Recognizing your wins along the way can boost your confidence and motivation to continue pushing forward.

8. **Stay Tenacious:** Perseverance is key when overcoming obstacles. Stay committed to your goals and keep moving forward, even when faced with setbacks or failures. Remember that setbacks are a natural part of the journey toward success.

Adopting a resilient mindset and implementing these tips can help you navigate any obstacles, carnivore or otherwise, with greater ease and confidence. Overcoming difficult challenges allows you to build evidence that you are a tenacious and ingenious person, capable of handling obstacles that come your way.

# 5

# OFF-BOARDING FROM A CARNIVORE DIET

After your 30-day carnivore boot camp, you have a decision to make. You may be so inspired by the results so far that you want to continue your new way of eating. On the other hand, you may have achieved the results you were looking for and feel ready to move forward with off-boarding from a carnivore diet. Or you might fall somewhere in between; you may have experienced some benefits from adhering to a meat-based approach but want to start incorporating some strategic plants back into your diet. Whichever path forward you choose, you will be able to take the principles and lessons learned from a carnivore way of eating with you.

## TRACKING YOUR PROGRESS

A great motivator when starting and completing any challenge is tracking the difference between your condition at the start and your state at the end of the challenge. While knowing you *feel* different at the end of the challenge is a powerful indicator of success, having objective measures in place that will show your progress can be even more rewarding. Having a record of how the challenge helped your move toward your goals can be a great motivator to reinitiate the challenge throughout your life as needed.

Tracking your progress is not just about the number on a scale. In some ways, the bathroom scale is a liar. It can't tell you that you are dehydrated, have better blood sugar levels, or lowered your cholesterol. While tracking weight is a great way to identify a general trend of weight loss or gain, it doesn't tell you whether that trend meets your body composition goals of building muscle or losing fat.

In addition to occasional weight tracking, I recommend using anthropometric measurements: body fat calipers that can be used to measure body fat versus lean mass, progress pictures that can show body composition like muscle growth in certain areas and fat loss in others, and how your clothes fit as your fat mass is being replaced by lean muscle.

In addition, if you have specific symptoms you are trying to correct, create a chart of the symptoms and rate them on a scale from 1 to 5, with 1 being no symptom present and 5 meaning the symptom is intolerable and needs to be treated by a health care provider. Weekly, and ideally at the same time of day during the same time of the week, rescore each of the symptoms. Very often, symptom reduction is gradual, and it can be difficult to objectively assess progress. By tracking the scale of your symptoms over time, it can show the progress you are making week to week, even if you don't feel different day to day.

### Symptom Scorecard

Using a symptom scorecard can help you understand the changes in your symptoms over time. This scorecard is based on the symptom clusters associated with Chronic Inflammatory Response Syndrome (CIRS), but you can modify it to track your unique symptoms.

## BEYOND THE 30-DAY CARNIVORE: EXTENDING YOUR PLAN

Typically, 30 days of carnivore is enough time to become fully adapted to your new way of eating. By the 30-day mark you should start seeing the benefits. If you have started to see some changes but haven't reached your goals yet, consider adding another 30 days. Especially if it took you a little while to adapt to your new way of eating, it can be helpful to adhere to your nutrition plan for a longer period of time to reap all the possible benefits from this diet strategy.

On the other hand, if you start seeing progress before the 30-day mark, you may feel inspired to continue with your new carnivore way of eating to see what additional benefits you might experience from another 30 days of eating a nutritionally dense diet.

Most carnivores peak, in terms of the observed benefits, at six to nine months of the diet. By six months, they have not only adapted, but their body has also had the time and energy it needs to heal. Some people choose to continue with a carnivore diet for months or even years after this point. Whether they appreciate the simple approach to optimal nutrition or rely on the diet for peak performance, plenty of people choose to stick to a meat-based diet long term.

Still, carnivore isn't a magic bullet for everything. If you initially get better with carnivore, and then get worse, or you follow the diet for six to nine months and are unable to resolve health concerns, you may need to dig a little deeper with your health care provider.

### Weight Management

If you started a carnivore diet to help with fat loss or muscle gain, hopefully you have seen signs of improvement by the end of your 30-day challenge. As I mentioned earlier, many new carnivores, especially those

# Symptom Scorecard

• • • • •

Score 1 to 5 on each symptom and track at regular intervals at the same time of day every time.

| SCORE DATE | 1 | 2 | 3 | 4 | 5 |
|---|---|---|---|---|---|
| Weak | | | | | |
| Hard to learn new things | | | | | |
| Aches | | | | | |
| Headaches | | | | | |
| Light sensitivity | | | | | |
| Memory impairment | | | | | |
| Hard to find words | | | | | |
| Joint pain | | | | | |
| Morning stiffness | | | | | |
| Shortness of breath | | | | | |
| Sinus congestion | | | | | |
| Appetite swings | | | | | |
| Poor temperature regulation | | | | | |
| Frequent urination | | | | | |
| Unusual skin sensitivity | | | | | |
| Tingling in extremities | | | | | |
| Abdominal pain | | | | | |

| SCORE DATE | 1 | 2 | 3 | 4 | 5 |
|---|---|---|---|---|---|
| Diarrhea | | | | | |
| Numbness | | | | | |
| Hard to concentrate | | | | | |
| Cough | | | | | |
| Excessive thirst | | | | | |
| Confusion | | | | | |
| Teary eyes | | | | | |
| Disorientation | | | | | |
| Metallic taste | | | | | |
| Red eyes | | | | | |
| Blurred vision | | | | | |
| Night sweats | | | | | |
| Mood swings | | | | | |
| Ice-pick pain | | | | | |
| Fatigue | | | | | |
| Static shocks | | | | | |
| Vertigo | | | | | |

transitioning from a typical diet full of seed oils and processed foods, experience a "whoosh" of weight loss.

This weight loss is typically from excess water being released as stored glucose is consumed for energy. Glucose is hydrophilic, meaning it holds onto water. After the initial water weight loss, most people experience a steady decline in weight as their body uses excess fat stores for energy. This typically occurs naturally, without tracking calories or macros. However, if you have a specific weight goal, you may find it beneficial to track your calorie intake.

Calorie targets are highly specific and depend on your height, weight, age, gender, activity level, and goals. There is no reason to ask for or chase after someone else's calorie goals. Instead, consider calculating your own using a TDEE calculator available online, my favorite is a carnivore calorie calculator built by a carnivore, available at https://criticalcarnivore.netlify.app.

It's helpful to use a carnivore-specific calorie calculator because many carnivores find they're able to eat more calories than they did on a standard American diet without increasing body weight. All calorie recommendations should be used as a guideline and recalibrated depending on your progress toward your goals.

## Macros

As a reminder, if you are coming to carnivore from a keto background, you may be surprised that keto macros are not the gold standard in the carnivore community. Macros are the categories of energy sources from food: carbohydrates, proteins, and fats. Keto is a macro diet, meaning the diet is centered around macro distribution goals. Carnivore is a food-source diet, meaning the diet is centered around nutrition source goals.

Finding the macro split of protein and fat that works best for you may take some trial and error. It is also highly dependent on your health goals. Typically, carnivores who are trying to heal fall on the higher end of the fat spectrum (80 percent or more of total calories from fat). Carnivores who are trying to lose weight and build lean muscle mass fall on the higher end of the protein spectrum (30 percent or more of total calories from protein). However, most carnivores find they naturally fall in a 20 to 30 percent protein and 70 to 80 percent fat macro split. Interestingly, the macro ratios found in eggs and the consumable meat of a cow both fall into the 30/70 macro split where 30 percent of the calories come from protein and 70 percent of the calories come from fat.

## Athletic Performance

If you tried a carnivore diet to help you improve athletic performance, you may want to stay on it. That's because your baseline performance can often be optimized by making small tweaks like adding carbs, experimenting with meal timings, or drinking electrolytes.

**Adding Carbs:** Glucose is the immediate energy used by the body in times of activity. If you train in high-intensity sports, you may find that adding some carbohydrates to your diet helps you feel more energized throughout your training. You can add carbohydrates through animal products, like milk, or consider adding unprocessed, least toxic fruits like oranges, avocados, or berries. Ideally, eating just ahead of your workout will help you utilize the glucose in your bloodstream and help manage any potential blood sugar spikes.

**Meal Timing:** If you are reluctant to add back carbs, look at changing your meal timings to better optimize your performance. There are some benefits to training fasted, like improved cortisol (stress hormone) baseline levels throughout the day, but a major downside is the extra burden of energy production in a fasted state. Consider eating just before your workout, leaving yourself enough time to digest, so that you have the most energy available right before your training.

**Drinking Electrolytes:** Electrolytes can help improve performance as they help with muscle contraction and nerve signaling. Additionally, electrolytes can help increase blood volume by changing your internal hydration balance. Drinking electrolytes just before or while working out can help optimize your performance by ensuring you have optimal electrolyte balance.

## Chronic Inflammatory Response Syndrome (CIRS)

Many in the carnivore community have found the root cause of their health issues to be chronic inflammatory response syndrome, or CIRS. CIRS happens when someone who is genetically predisposed to difficulty in eliminating a biotoxin encounters that biotoxin. So far, some of the biotoxins identified by CIRS researchers include mold, Lyme, pfiesteria, and toxic algae.

If you are experiencing stubborn weight loss, hair loss, muscle cramping, plantar fasciitis, nighttime urination, residual autoimmune or other health issues after pursuing carnivore for six to nine months, it may be a sign you have CIRS.

## Underlying Issues and Co-Infections

Regardless of whether your carnivore journey leads you to a CIRS diagnosis, you may find that it reveals a health baseline that still has issues. If you are still experiencing symptoms after trying carnivore, it is worth pursuing a root-cause diagnosis. For many people who have lived in a malnourished state for the majority of their lives, they may find that their less-than-optimal immune function has opened the door to co-infections.

Common co-infections are small intestinal bacteria overgrowth (SIBO), candida (yeast), and *H. pylori*, a common intestinal bacterial infection. These can all impact your gastrointestinal health. While carnivore may help better manage the symptoms of these co-infections, they may not ultimately eliminate the underlying infection. Work with your health care practitioner to properly eliminate co-infections like these.

### Carnivore Detox

If you choose to continue with a carnivore diet, you can add other complementary lifestyle changes to further optimize your health. Removing toxins from your system is a great place to start.

We are an ancient species living in a modern world and our exposure to toxins in our environment is unprecedented. While toxins can include the chemicals found in our household cleaners and personal products, they can also be found in the media we consume, the people we surround ourselves with, and the thoughts that fill our every waking moment. Here are some ways you can detox:

- Unsubscribe from junk emails

- Leave toxic relationships

- Avoid toxic media

- Unfollow social media that makes you feel less-than

- Retrain negative thought patterns

- Filter your tap water

- Buy organic food

- Use natural products

## OFF-BOARDING OPTIONS

Long term, you may choose not to adhere strictly to a carnivore way of eating. You may decide to reintroduce some foods, or you may choose to leverage carnivore cyclically, as you need it. Regardless of how you plan your nutrition moving forward, it can be helpful to understand your options and how to approach them.

### Reintroducing Plant Foods

If you choose to reintroduce plant foods moving forward, there are two typical approaches you could take: ketovore or animal-based. Ketovore is a keto-focused approach to plant reintroductions, whereas proponents of the animal-based diet support a more "ancestral" approach to carb-incorporation. Depending on your lifestyle, your health history, and your goals, one approach may feel more applicable to you than the other. You do not have to reintroduce anything if you do not want to, but it can be helpful to know that the option is available to you, if and when you are ready to take it.

**Switching to Ketovore:** If you find ketogenic macros helpful, you may want to approach reintroductions through a ketovore lens. A ketovore diet is a specialized form of the ketogenic diet that emphasizes primarily consuming animal-based foods, particularly those high in fat and protein, while continuing to limit plant-based foods. This approach focuses on reintroducing plant foods that align with the macronutrient requirements of a ketogenic diet.

One way to look at reintroducing plant foods on a ketovore diet is as a flavor modifier, rather than a main part of the meal. For example, using a couple tablespoons of diced onion, a clove of garlic, and a tablespoon of tomato paste with chicken broth to make a Bolognese sauce with ground beef would be a ketovore approach that emphasizes the meat for nutrition and the plant foods for flavor. Think of it as "How little plant matter can I get away with?" rather than "How much plant matter can I get away with?" It can be helpful to remember how good you felt without eating plants. The goal of ketovore is to retain the benefits of being meat-based while adding plants for variety and flavor.

### Common Ketovore Plant Foods for Reintroduction

- Cruciferous vegetables like broccoli and cauliflower, which are relatively low in carbs and can be consumed in small portions.

- Avocado, a high-fat fruit that is low in net carbs and rich in fiber, making it a popular choice for ketovore dieters.

- Olives and olive oil, providing healthy fats and minimal carbohydrates.

- Coconut and coconut products, including coconut oil, coconut milk, and shredded coconut, which are low in carbs and high in healthy fats.

- Nuts and seeds like macadamia nuts, pecans, and cashews, which are low in net carbs and high in fats and fiber.

- Berries such as strawberries, raspberries, and blackberries, which are lower in sugar compared to other fruits and can be consumed in small quantities.

- Non-starchy vegetables like bell peppers, zucchini, and cucumber, which provide some vitamins and minerals while being relatively low in carbohydrates.

- Mushrooms, which are low in carbs and can be incorporated into various dishes for flavor and texture.

- Herbs and spices such as basil, cilantro, and turmeric, which add flavor to meals without significantly increasing carbohydrate intake.

### Switching to Animal-Based

The other lens to view plant reintroduction is from an animal-based diet perspective.

### Keto Diet: Net Carbs vs. Total Carbs

Some keto dieters track net carbs, or the total carbs less any fiber or sugar alcohols on the nutritional label, as they claim those carbs are not digested so should not be counted. But tracking total carbs instead of net carbs on a keto diet means you're keeping tabs on all carbs in your food, including fiber and sugar alcohols. It's like having the full picture of what you're eating rather than just part of it. Tracking total carbs allows you to enjoy your chosen plant foods without gaslighting yourself about how much plant matter you are really eating.

An animal-based diet still emphasizes meat as the foundation to nutrition, but rather than focusing on adding plants that contribute to a macronutrient goal, it emphasizes plants thought to be aligned with ancestral eating practices. Plant toxins are typically stored in the roots, stems, leaves, and seeds of plants, as these are the parts of plants needed to sustain life and reproduce.

Fruit, however, is designed by plants to be eaten. Fruit typically contains the seed of the plant. Once animals digest fruit and evacuate, the seeds disperse and proliferate. Animal-based dieters recognize fruit as the least-toxic plant foods and therefore the most beneficial to reincorporate into your diet.

### Common Low-Toxin Plant Foods for Animal-Based Reintroduction:

- Avocado is a high-fat fruit that is low in toxins and therefore popular with animal-based dieters.

- Berries are also said to contain low amounts of plant toxins.

- Squash, as the vehicle for the plant's seeds, is also deemed least toxic by people who follow an animal-based way of eating.

- Cucumbers (with skin and seeds removed) and other melons also produce less plant toxins according to these dieters.

- Fruits like apples, oranges, bananas, pineapple, mangoes, and peaches are on the animal-based "safe" list.

- Olives are another high-fat fruit commonly incorporated into animal-based diets.

- Dates are considered least toxic fruits.

- Honey, while not a plant and not an animal, is specifically and commonly included in this way of eating.

## Beware of Plant Toxins and Fructose

When reintroducing plant foods in the animal-based diet, consider not just the amount of plants you are eating, but also the amount of any one plant toxin you are eating. Eating a variety of "least toxic" plant foods can help you avoid the overaccumulation of any one plant toxin.

On the other hand, most of the "least toxic" plant foods recommended by animal-based dieters are high in fructose. Fructose is one of the three monosaccharides (sugars) found in nature along with glucose and lactose. This sugar is commonly found in fruits, but also honey. However, fructose is structurally different from glucose and lactose, and may have negative effects on metabolism.

Many people are familiar with lactose intolerance, or the inability to digest lactose, the sugar found in milk and other dairy products, but few may be aware of fructose intolerance.[90] Fructose intolerance, also known as fructose malabsorption or fructose sensitivity, is a condition characterized by difficulty digesting and absorbing fructose. If you have fructose intolerance, you lack the necessary enzymes to efficiently break down fructose in the small intestine,

## Avocados: Friend or Foe?

While animal-based dieters claim that avocado is a fruit and therefore lower in toxins and safe to eat, they may fail to mention the presence of persin, a fungicidal plant toxin present in the pit and skin of the plant that leaches, in low concentrations, into the avocado flesh. While persin appears "safe" in moderate amounts, persin toxicity can cause cardiac issues and trouble breathing, so monitor your intake accordingly.

## Improved Lactose Tolerance

An interesting anecdotal benefit reported in the Harvard Carnivore Study was that some respondents, after following a strict carnivore diet for a couple months, found that they were no longer lactose intolerant. If you avoid dairy due to lactose intolerance, you may be able to reintroduce it after adhering to a carnivore diet to no ill effect.

While the mechanism for carnivore correcting lactose intolerance is unknown, lactase, the enzyme responsible for breaking down lactose, is a protein made out of amino acids that are found in meat. If your lactose intolerance is due to not having enough essential amino acids to build lactase efficiently, eating a nutritionally dense carnivore diet may correct your lactose intolerance. If your lactose intolerance is due to genetic or other reasons, you may retain lactose intolerance after trying a carnivore diet.

leading to symptoms such as abdominal pain, bloating, diarrhea, and gas after consuming foods high in fructose. Fructose intolerance can also lead to nutritional deficiencies as it interrupts typical digestion.

Another possible concern from eating a diet high in fructose is fatty liver disease. The body stores excess fructose in the liver, and if you consume too much fructose, it converts to fat in the liver. There are two main types: non-alcoholic fatty liver disease (NAFLD), which is linked to factors such as obesity, insulin resistance, and metabolic syndrome, and alcoholic fatty liver disease (AFLD), which is caused by excessive alcohol consumption. Eating too much fructose, especially in the context of a high-fat diet, can lead to NAFLD.[91] Fatty liver disease can lead to complications like liver cirrhosis, liver cancer, and cardiac disease. Work with your health care provider to monitor your liver and overall health to prevent serious health complications.

## CYCLING ON AND OFF THE DIET

Once you have tried carnivore for 30 days, and you experience some of the potential benefits many people experience through this way of eating, you may not want to continue the diet, and that is okay! You may find that the flavor, variety, and convenience plant foods provide, for you, outweigh the health benefits you glean from a meat-based way of eating. However, once you have seen what a carnivore way of eating can do to help you reach your goals, you may want to return to it cyclically to "reset" your physical health, mental health, or fitness baseline.

A cyclical carnivore diet is one that is adhered to, strictly, for a limited period of time, and repeated at a predetermined or as-needed frequency to positively impact your health or fitness outcomes. Some people choose to do a month of carnivore yearly, as a way to "reset" their nutritional status. Commonly, this is done in January, World Carnivore Month, as popularized by podcast host Joe Rogan.

### Carnivore as a Diet Reset

Some cycle back to carnivore after the holidays as a "diet reset" to help recalibrate hunger and satiety signals, especially after indulging in lots of holiday carbs. The weight loss, improved energy, and sense of well-being that carnivore can help you achieve are an excellent way to start the year. You can always return to a carnivore way of eating, as needed, to reconnect with the positive benefits of eating a nutritionally dense diet.

### Carnivore as a Health Reset

Another reason to restart the 30-day carnivore boot camp is if you experienced positive health outcomes from the first 30 days and want to regain some of that symptom relief. However, it should be noted that if a carnivore diet is required for you to alleviate your symptoms, then carnivore is a band-aid, not a solution. A repeated need to pursue carnivore in order to feel okay is a good indicator that root-cause healing is needed.

## CARNIVORE IS A DIET, NOT AN IDENTITY

At the end of the day, a carnivore way of eating is a diet, a tool in your nutritional arsenal that you can use to help you achieve your best possible self. A carnivore diet can support your bigger life goals by providing you with a nutrient-dense foundation that allows you to perform at your best. When your diet allows you to feel your best, you can show up in your life as the best version of you!

Carnivore is meant to support your identity by helping you achieve your dreams. Your way of eating—whether it is a carnivore diet, a plant-based diet, or a standard American diet—is just that: a diet. It is not your identity and should not be pursued for its own sake.

A diet should be pursued for the results it gives you—for how it makes you feel and supports your bigger life goals. At any point in your health journey, if you feel that a carnivore diet is no longer supporting your ultimate health baseline, it is okay to pursue other nutritional strategies.

# CONCLUSION

## A NEW WAY OF EATING, A NEW LIFE

**Congratulations!** By reading this book, you have taken the first step on your new journey. No matter where you go from here, I hope you feel more knowledgeable and empowered to make good decisions for better health. You may, as many have, find that the 30-day carnivore boot camp has impacted your life in unexpected ways that last well beyond a month of dietary changes. For many of the people I coach, they find carnivore gives them the confidence they need to pursue big life goals. It has been an incredible gift to watch fellow carnivores regain their health, discover root-cause issues that they could pursue treatment for, break free from the confines of mental health disorders, lose body fat, and achieve fitness goals they never thought were possible for them.

At the end of the day, we are all different; we all have different health histories, lifestyles, and goals. So, it's impossible to create a one-size-fits-all guide for any lifestyle choice. Your experience with carnivore may lead you down a different path than mine did. For me, carnivore became a gateway to improved physical and emotional health.

For you, carnivore may be a tool you keep in your back pocket when you need a reset of your health or fitness.

### BECOMING YOUR BEST SELF

One of the most inspiring changes I have seen in many carnivores is the newfound sense of themselves. Distilling your diet, and many things in your life, to the most essential parts has a way of opening space for clarity. While it is easy to sing the praises of the health and fitness gains of a carnivore way of eating, it is much harder to describe and explain the confidence and self-esteem gained. In reflection, I think part of this confidence stems from the simple step of choosing to eat this way for yourself. In our modern, fast-paced, success-focused world, choosing yourself and your health is a radical act.

One of the biggest lessons I learned on my carnivore journey was that taking care of myself and my health is the least selfish thing I can do. My family, my friends, and the people impacted by my life deserve the best of what I have to give. The only way that I can give the best of myself is to be my best self. That is what I hope my book has offered you: a diet structure that you can use as a tool to actualize the best version of you. We are offered many things in the smorgasbord of life, from tools to help us grow to coping mechanisms like bingeing television and processed foods to numb the dread of change. We can easily choose to become comfortable in the uncomfortable but familiar. Whether or not you choose to go carnivore, I hope that I've inspired you to choose yourself, your dreams, and a well-lived life.

## NAVIGATING CARNIVORE INFORMATION ON SOCIAL MEDIA

If you're interested in making carnivore a lifestyle choice, as I have, tread carefully as you explore this topic on social media. Influencers have a weird dilemma because each new post antiquates the last. It's difficult to produce content in a niche where very little new information is coming out. This makes social media an echo chamber. One piece of information is latched onto, reproduced, and regurgitated until the original content has lost its original intention. To complicate things even further, some influencers contort and distort information to monetize it, even making people fearful so they'll buy their product.

When looking into new carnivore concepts and ideas, first ask: Does this information feel true for me? Is a promo code or sponsorship motivating this person to push this idea? What research can I do before I make a good decision? Even if, through your research, you find that this new information is accurate, you will need to question how it applies to your own life. Does it make sense for you, your health history, and your goals? If it doesn't, there is no need to implement it. Focus on the strategies that make you feel your best; the rest is clutter!

Doctors who work with patients are held to a very high standard by state medical boards, but there are no checks and balances in the online carnivore community. We're lucky to have several doctors in our community who contribute valuable content. Content from doctors is assumed to be correct and legitimate, but this doesn't mean that all content from a "medical" source is right for you or that all content is factual. It may, in fact, cause harm. My advice? Follow the same guidelines as you would with any other influencer to assess whether the information is true and whether it is applicable to you.

Just as individual influencers can create trends in the carnivore space, so can communities. As you go along your carnivore journey, you may notice groups of people participating in challenges to give up dairy, coffee, or salt; to restrict their diets to only ruminants; or to walk 10,000 steps per day. None of these trends is inherently or universally bad, but it is important for you to assess whether they may be bad for you before you join in. For example, if you just started a new job, especially if it's physically taxing, and you are trying to add in 10,000 extra steps per day, while objectively a good health choice for many, it may not be a good health choice for you.

Being a carnivore means that you are a person who is willing to march to the beat of a different drum for your own health. Keep marching along your path, and don't worry about the beat someone else is jamming to.

For additional recipes and carnivore meal inspiration, follow me at:

*www.instagram.com/ladycarnivory*
*www.ladycarnivory.com*

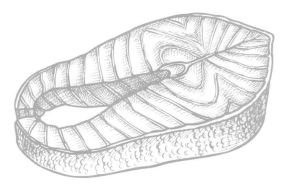

# APPENDIX

## FORMS OF MAGNESIUM

Magnesium is an essential mineral, one of many eletrolytes needed to transport electrical signals throughout the body. It's also involved in many physiological processes. As a supplement, it is often paired with other compounds to improve bioavailability and to leverage specific benefits of magnesium. Different forms of magnesium offer varying benefits and have different considerations for their use. Here's a breakdown of some common forms of magnesium and their benefits.

### Magnesium Citrate

**Benefits**: Magnesium citrate is one of the most bioavailable forms of magnesium, meaning the body readily absorbs it. It has a laxative effect and is often used to support digestive health and alleviate constipation. Magnesium citrate may also help improve sleep quality.

**Considerations:** The laxative effect of magnesium citrate that can be helpful for those experiencing constipation may be too strong for others. Start with a lower dose and titrate up as needed until you are at the full dose as listed by the supplement packaging. Another consideration is that citric acid is commercially produced by processing black mold, so those sensitive to mold may want to avoid this form of magnesium.

### Magnesium Glycinate

**Benefits:** If you are looking for a bioavailable form of magnesium without the laxative effect, magnesium glycinate is less likely to cause digestive upset compared to magnesium citrate. This form is well-absorbed and may especially support relaxation, stress relief, and improved sleep quality. Magnesium glycinate is a better option for individuals with sensitive stomachs.

**Considerations:** Magnesium glycinate is generally well-tolerated, but some people may experience mild gastrointestinal discomfort at higher doses. Make sure you adhere to the package instructions to avoid negative impact.

### Magnesium Oxide

**Benefits:** A less bioavailable form of magnesium, meaning it is less well-utilized by the body, is magnesium oxide. This form has a high magnesium content but, because of its pairing with oxide, it is less well-absorbed by the body. It can be used as a gentle laxative, especially for those with sensitive stomachs.

**Considerations:** Since it is not absorbed as well, magnesium oxide may provide less benefit overall compared to other forms. Even though it has a gentler laxative effect, those with sensitive gastrointestinal systems may still find it difficult to tolerate.

## Magnesium Chloride

**Benefits:** Magnesium chloride is a highly absorbable form of magnesium and can be absorbed through the skin. As such, it is often used topically, including as magnesium oil or bath salts. Magnesium chloride may help reduce muscle tension, promote relaxation, and support exercise recovery.

**Considerations:** Oral supplementation of this form of magnesium is uncommon due to its limited availability as an oral supplement. However, powder and pill versions of magnesium chloride can be found online.

## Magnesium Threonate

**Benefits:** Magnesium threonate is specifically designed to penetrate the blood-brain barrier more effectively than other forms. It has potential cognitive benefits such as improved memory, cognitive function, and mood support. This form may also support overall neurological health and cognitive function.

**Considerations:** A newer form of magnesium, magnesium threonate is promising. But because it is more specialized, it may be less widely available on the market and is also typically the most expensive form of magnesium.

## Magnesium Malate

**Benefits:** Magnesium malate is a combination of magnesium and malic acid. Naturally found in fruits, malic acid promotes the production of energy in the body, so magnesium malate is a popular choice for reducing fatigue and supporting energy levels. This form may also help alleviate muscle pain, supporting exercise recovery and reducing muscle aches for individuals with conditions like fibromyalgia.

**Considerations:** Magnesium malate has good bioavailability and is generally well-tolerated, even for those with sensitive stomachs. Since it is combined with a substantial amount of malic acid, it may not provide as high a magnesium content per dose as other forms.

## Magnesium Sulfate (Epsom Salt)

**Benefits:** Magnesium sulfate, or Epsom salt, is a common ingredient in bath salts and is known for its muscle-relaxing and stress-relieving benefits. Dissolving this form in warm water can soothe sore muscles and promote relaxation.

**Considerations:** Aside from being used as a bath salt, magnesium sulfate is a powerful laxative. Oral supplementation is not recommended outside of medical uses.

# Sample Schedule for Intermittent Fasting

## 8-HOUR EATING WINDOW
### (11:00 am to 7:00 pm)

**6:00 am** .............. Wake up (morning supplements)

**6:15 am** .............. Fasted workout (to leverage weight loss and reduced cortisol baseline)

**9:00 am** .............. Fatty coffee (see page 95)

**11:00 am** ........... First meal/breakfast

**1:00 pm** .............. Electrolyte drink (see page 97)

**3:00 pm** .............. Second meal/lunch

**6:00 pm** .............. Third meal/dinner (evening supplements, if they need to be taken with food)

**10:00 pm** ........... Bed time

• • • • •

## 6-HOUR EATING WINDOW
### (12:00 pm to 6:00 pm)

**6:00 am** .............. Wake up (morning supplements)

**6:15 am** .............. Fasted workout (to leverage weight loss and reduced cortisol baseline)

**9:00 am** .............. Fatty coffee (see page 95)

**12:00 pm** ........... First meal/breakfast

**1:00 pm** .............. Electrolyte drink (see page 97)

**3:00 pm** .............. Second meal/lunch

**5:00 pm** .............. Third meal/dinner (evening supplements, if they need to be taken with food)

**10:00 pm** ........... Bed time

## OXALATE CHEAT SHEET

In her book *Toxic Superfoods: How Oxalate Overload Is Making You Sick—and How to Get Better*, oxalate expert Sally K. Norton discusses the issue of oxalate accumulation and dumping. Oxalic acid, present in plants, binds with calcium in the human body, creating oxalate crystals. These crystals accumulate in tissues of the body, including joints, kidneys, and other soft tissues. Oxalate accumulation can cause the symptoms of many chronic illnesses, and reducing oxalate consumption can alleviate the presentation of many common maladies such as plantar fasciitis, joint pain, digestive issues, and skin conditions.

While eliminating oxalates can alleviate inflammation and symptoms associated with the accumulation of oxalates, when you completely eliminate oxalates, you may experience a phenomenon known as "oxalate dumping." Oxalate dumping is when your body starts excreting oxalates and can present as grainy tears, cloudy urine, or even skin lesions that excrete these salty oxalate crystals. To avoid extreme symptoms of oxalate dumping, microdosing oxalate-containing foods can slow down the excretion process.

Removing oxalate-rich foods from your diet can help alleviate these common symptoms and expedite your healing.

### Some Foods High in Oxalate

- Tea (while not particularly high in oxalate, it is a highly soluble form)
- Almonds
- Spinach and swiss chard
- Beets
- Peanuts
- Soy
- Chocolate and cocoa
- Whole grains like wheat and bran

you are experiencing frequent constipation or diarrhea past the adaptation phase of carnivore, it may be a sign of underlying health issues that need to be addressed. Paying attention to your bowel movement frequency, texture, and color can help you identify levers for root cause healing.

Work with an appropriate practitioner to resolve the root-cause issue causing gastrointestinal issues.

## BOWEL MOVEMENT GUIDE

Your digestive system is an excellent indicator of your overall health. Your bowel movements should be regular, easy, relatively solid, and medium-dark in color. If

### Diarrhea or Loose Stools

Loose stools can indicate gastrointestinal issues like parasites; bacterial, fungal, or yeast overgrowth; chronic inflammation leading to leaky gut or irritable bowel syndrome; or autoimmune dysfunction.

## The Bristol Stool Scale

The Bristol Stool Scale is a helpful way to describe your bowel movements to your doctor without needing to bring in a sample. Developed by researchers with the help of sixty-six volunteers, they were able to categorize and describe different bowel movements.

- Type 1: separate hard lumps, like nuts, that are hard to pass

- Type 2: sausage-shaped but lumpy

- Type 3: sausage-shaped but with cracks on the surface

- Type 4: sausage or snake-like, smooth and soft

- Type 5: soft blobs with clear-cut edges that are easy to pass

- Type 6: fluffy pieces with ragged edges, mushy

- Type 7: watery, no solid pieces, entirely liquid

Generally, the ideal stool is type 3 or 4, which should pass easily without being watery. Type 1 or 2 stool is considered constipation. If you have type 5, 6, or 7, you are likely experiencing diarrhea.

Source: Lewis SJ, Heaton KW. Stool form scale as a useful guide to intestinal transit time. Scand J Gastroenterol. 1997 Sep;32(9):920-4. doi: 10.3109/00365529709011203. PMID: 9299672.

### Constipation

Hard to pass or infrequent stools are signs of low gut motility, or movement. This can be caused by inflammation or certain auto-immune conditions, or as a side effect to certain medications and stress.

### Green-colored Stool

Green stool can indicate the presence of undigested bile, which can indicate food is being digested too quickly, so that the bile is not able to break down dietary fat and be absorbed into the intestine. Poor bile absorption can indicate issues with detox pathways as the liver over-produces bile acids.

### Clay-colored Stool

Clay-colored stool may indicate low bile acid production, which can indicate issues with the gallbladder. The gallbladder works like a muscle—you have to use it, or you will lose optimal function. So if you are coming to carnivore from a low-fat diet, it may take a while for your gallbladder to adapt bile production to the higher fat intake. Ox bile supplements can help the adaptation process, but long-term need for these supplements may indicate an underlying issue with your gallbladder.

### Black-colored Stool

Stool that is black in color may indicate the presence of blood in your intestines. This is common in some autoimmune conditions like Crohn's disease, but can also be indicative of bacterial, fungal, or yeast infection.

# CHEAT SHEET
## Beef Cuts

When I first started eating a carnivore diet, I was overwhelmed by the different cuts of beef. It took me a while to understand which cuts I liked best and how to cook them optimally. Below is an overview of common beef cuts, their characteristics, and ideal cooking methods.

### RIBEYE STEAK

Ribeyes are cut from the rib section of the cow. This cut is fatty, well-marbled, tender, and flavorful. A true favorite in the carnivore community!

**How to Cook:** This cut is best suited for hot and fast cooking methods like grilling, pan-searing, or broiling.

### FILET MIGNON

Filet mignon is also known as tenderloin steak as it comes from the tenderloin muscle. It is exceptionally tender but is on the leaner side with minimal fat marbling.

**How to Cook:** Filet mignon is another cut well-suited to hot and fast cooking such as pan-searing, grilling, or roasting.

### NEW YORK STRIP STEAK

New York strip is cut from the short loin. This steak is moderately tender with a good balance of flavor and tenderness. New York strip typically has a strip of fat down the long edge of the steak that is best when well-seared on high-heat.

**How to Cook:** Best suited for grilling, pan-searing, or broiling.

### T-BONE STEAK

The T-bone steak is named for its T-shaped bone. This steak contains both the strip loin and tenderloin muscles on either side of the bone. It has a delightful combination of tenderness and flavor.

**How to Cook:** Best suited for grilling, pan-searing, or broiling.

### SIRLOIN STEAK

This steak is cut from the sirloin section of the cow. Sirloin steak is leaner than cuts from the rib or loin and less tender.

**How to Cook:** Best suited for grilling, pan-searing, or broiling. Cook to medium or medium-rare to avoid a too-tough steak.

### FLANK STEAK

This steak comes from the abdominal muscles of the cow and is lean and super flavorful but tends to be less tender than other cuts.

**How to Cook:** Best suited for broiling or grilling quickly at high heat.

## SKIRT STEAK

Skirt steak is similar to flank steak but comes from the diaphragm muscles of the cow, rather than the abdominal muscles. It is lean and flavorful, and has a coarse texture well- suited to being cut into strips—like for fajitas.

**How to Cook:** Best suited for broiling or grilling quickly at high heat.

## CHUCK ROAST

Chuck roast is cut from the shoulder area of the cow. Well-marbled and flavorful, this cut is typically slow-cooked to tenderize the tough connective tissues.

**How to Cook:** Best suited for braising, slow-roasting, or stewing.

## BRISKET

A popular cut found at barbecue joints, brisket comes from the chest area of the cow. This cut is known for its tender texture and rich flavor when cooked low and slow.

**How to Cook:** Best suited for braising, slow-roasting, or smoking.

## SHORT RIBS

This cut is from the rib section of the cow and contains layers of meat and fat. Short ribs, when cooked low and slow, result in rich flavor and tender texture.

**How to Cook:** Best suited for braising, slow-cooking, or smoking.

## PRIME RIB

Also known as standing rib roast, this is cut from the rib primal section of the cow and is well-marbled, flavorful, and tender.

**How to Cook:** Prime rib is ideally cooked initially at a high heat to sear the outside of the roast, then slow-roasting at a lower temperature until tender.

## TOP ROUND ROAST

Top round roast comes from the round primal section of the cow and is lean with minimal marbling. It is typically less tender than other roast cuts, so it needs to be slow roasted. When cooked correctly, it has rich flavor.

**How to Cook:** Best suited for roasting low and slow, then slicing thinly against the grain for tender bites.

## BOTTOM ROUND ROAST

This roast, also known as rump roast, comes from the round primal section of the cow. Bottom round roast is lean and has moderate fat marbling. While it is less tender, it does have good beefy flavor.

**How to Cook:** Best suited for roasting low and slow, braising, or cooking in a slow cooker for tenderness.

## EYE OF ROUND ROAST

This roast is a lean cut that comes from the round primal of the cow. It is relatively tender compared to other round roasts. It has minimal fat marbling and so is best cooked rare to medium-rare.

**How to Cook:** This cut is best suited for roasting low and slow, then slicing thinly against the grain for tenderness.

## CROSS RIB ROAST

Cross rib roast comes from the chuck primal section of the cow. It is well-marbled, flavorful, and relatively tender. A versatile cut, it can be cooked using various methods, making it an easy and delightful roast to cook.

**How to Cook:** Best suited for roasting, braising, or slow-cooking for tenderness.

## TRI-TIP ROAST

This roast comes from the bottom sirloin primal section of the cow. It has a triangular shape, inspiring the name. It is well-marbled, flavorful, and has a tender texture if cooked properly.

**How to Cook:** Best suited for grilling, smoking, or roasting, slicing thinly against the grain for tenderness.

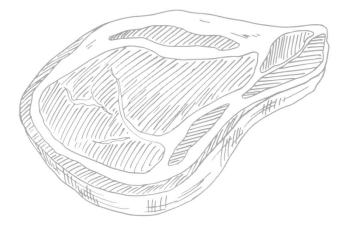

## SAMPLE MEAL PLAN FOR CHRONIC ILLNESS (PAGE 160)

For many people starting a carnivore diet, it is best to focus on keeping the diet easy and interesting to promote adherence. This can look like incorporating limited seasonings or dairy products like cheese for added variety. However, people who are pursuing a carnivore diet to eliminate symptoms associated with chronic illness may want to take a more strict approach to avoid histamines, focusing on higher-quality, unaged meat. Additionally, it can be helpful to eliminate dairy and eggs, as they are possibly inflammatory. Finally, focusing on added fat can help you leverage the benefits of ketogenic macros, which have been shown to have a therapeutic effect on inflammation. Whole meat, cooked to doneness, for each and every meal is both accessible and nutritious for those eating carnivore to heal.

## SAMPLE MEAL PLAN FOR KETOGENIC MACROS (PAGE 161)

Many people come to carnivore from a ketogenic diet, which is a macro-focused diet, requiring the adherents to eat 80 percent of their calories from fat and 20 percent of their calories from protein. As previously discussed, ketogenic macros have been shown to have therapeutic effects on inflammation and also contribute to fat loss. Since a ketogenic diet is characterized by its macronutrient composition and not the food composition, it is possible to combine the macro-approach to eating with a carnivore diet. To properly leverage ketogenic macros on a carnivore diet, you may need to add more fat to your meat from butter, tallow (beef fat), duck fat, ghee (clarified butter), schmalz (chicken fat), or lard (pork fat).

# SAMPLE MEAL PLAN FOR CHRONIC ILLNESS

## SUNDAY

✓ **BREAKFAST**
Air-Fryer Steak Bites
(page 82)

✓ **LUNCH**
Pan-cooked ground lamb

✓ **DINNER**
Roasted Chicken Thighs
(page 88)

## MONDAY

✓ **BREAKFAST**
Roasted Chicken Thighs
(page 88)

✓ **LUNCH**
Oven-Baked Salmon Bites
(page 80)

✓ **DINNER**
Cooked Ground Beef
Patties (without cheese,
page 87)

## TUESDAY

✓ **BREAKFAST**
Roasted Pork Ribs
(page 89)

✓ **LUNCH**
Pan-cooked ground lamb

✓ **DINNER**
Air-Fryer Steak Bites
(page 82)

## WEDNESDAY

✓ **BREAKFAST**
Roasted Chicken Thighs
(page 88)

✓ **LUNCH**
Oven-Baked Salmon
Bites (page 80)

✓ **DINNER**
Cooked Ground Beef
Patties (without cheese,
page 87)

## THURSDAY

✓ **BREAKFAST**
Roasted Pork Ribs
(page 89)

✓ **LUNCH**
Roasted Chicken Thighs
(page 88)

✓ **DINNER**
Oven-Baked Salmon
Bites (page 80)

## FRIDAY

✓ **BREAKFAST**
Cooked Ground Beef
Patties (without cheese,
page 87)

✓ **LUNCH**
Roasted Pork Ribs
(page 89)

✓ **DINNER**
Air-Fryer Steak Bites
(page 82)

## SATURDAY

✓ **BREAKFAST**
Roasted Chicken Thighs
(page 88)

✓ **LUNCH**
Oven-Baked Salmon
Bites (page 80)

✓ **DINNER**
Cooked Ground Beef
Patties (without cheese,
page 87)

# SAMPLE MEAL PLAN FOR KETOGENIC MACROS

## SUNDAY

✓ **BREAKFAST**
Make-Ahead Meaty Breakfast Muffins (page 74)

✓ **LUNCH**
Chili (page 85) topped with cheese

✓ **DINNER**
Parmesan Pork Chop Bites (page 86)

## MONDAY

✓ **BREAKFAST**
Easy Cheesy Breakfast Taco (page 73) and Fatty Coffee (page 95)

✓ **LUNCH**
Prep-Friendly Pork Enchiladas (page 81) with extra cheese

✓ **DINNER**
Roasted Chicken Thighs (page 88) with added butter

## TUESDAY

✓ **BREAKFAST**
Deviled Eggs (page 75) with Fatty Coffee (page 95)

✓ **LUNCH**
Cheesy Chicken Casserole (page 84)

✓ **DINNER**
Cooked Ground Beef Patties with Cheese (page 87)

## WEDNESDAY

✓ **BREAKFAST**
French Slow Scramble (page 76) with Fatty Coffee (page 95)

✓ **LUNCH**
Parmesan Pork Chop Bites (page 86)

✓ **DINNER**
Cooked Ground Beef Patties (without cheese, page 87)

## THURSDAY

✓ **BREAKFAST**
Breakfast Casserole (page 77) and Fatty Coffee (page 95)

✓ **LUNCH**
Roasted Pork Ribs (page 89) with added butter

✓ **DINNER**
Oven-Baked Salmon Bites (page 80) with added butter

## FRIDAY

✓ **BREAKFAST**
Egg Wrap Burrito (page 78) with Fatty Coffee (page 95)

✓ **LUNCH**
Chicken Cordon Bleu Loaf (page 83)

✓ **DINNER**
Air-Fryer Steak Bites (page 82) with added butter

## SATURDAY

✓ **BREAKFAST**
Breakfast Scramble (page 79) and Fatty Coffee (page 95)

✓ **LUNCH**
Prep-Friendly Pork Enchiladas (page 81)

✓ **DINNER**
Cheesy Chicken Casserole (page 84)

# ABOUT THE AUTHOR

**JACIE GREGORY** is an enthusiastic carnivore and CIRS educator. She loves creating content that makes science understandable and progress toward health goals more accessible. She is best known for her creative carnivore recipes that make the diet practical and fun. She is less well-known for but equally passionate about mindset management: a limbic retraining practice that supports better health by helping to regulate the nervous system.

Born in southern California, and raised in Tucson, Arizona, she spent the early years of her young adult life struggling with chronic health issues like Obsessive Compulsive Disorder, eating disorders, and low-grade joint pain. After learning about fitness competitions through creators on YouTube, she became inspired to unlock her best health so that she could one day compete too.

Jacie moved to Denver, Colorado as a young adult and fell in love with the mountains, and shockingly, the snow! Living in an active community, her interest in health and fitness grew, leading her to try many different nutritional strategies until she stumbled upon a carnivore diet. The health gains she achieved through this way of eating inspired her to share her journey on social media, become a carnivore coach, and eventually obtain a nutrition coaching certification through the National Academy of Sports Medicine. Her health improvements were so profound that she did achieve her long-harbored goal of competing in a fitness competition in the summer of 2021.

After falling ill from biotoxin exposure, her passion for carnivore and its antiinflammatory properties expanded. She learned about healing from the biotoxin illness called Chronic Inflammatory Response Syndrome (CIRS) through the Shoemaker Protocol, and created a community for people healing from the same illness. She is also a CIRS educator, teaching people about the illness and how to recover from it through social media graphics and a weekly podcast.

Outside of her work in online health communities, Jacie enjoys spending time outdoors with her dogs, Emma and Murphy. She often travels and loves connecting with new people in new places. Her favorite pastime is exploring creativity through many mediums, like recipe creation, writing, and aesthetic design. When she isn't traveling or testing new recipes, you can find her eating her favorite meal —eggs and bacon—while snuggled up watching scary movies with her dogs.

Through her work online, Jacie coaches individuals to help them achieve root-cause healing through nutritional strategies, mindset practices, and other modalities. She believes that when we take excellent care of ourselves, we show up for our friends and family as the best version of ourselves. And when we are the best versions of ourselves, we can do our best work in the world.

# ACKNOWLEDGMENTS

First and foremost, I would like to express my deepest gratitude to my mom. Your unwavering belief in me has been my life-long guiding light. Your love and support have been the foundation upon which I have built my dreams.

Lawrence Nimbach, thank you for always allowing me to come home. Your generosity has been immeasurable, and I am deeply grateful for your kindness and support.

Dr. Shawn Baker, your advocacy for the carnivore diet and your bravery in sharing your personal experiences have been a source of immense inspiration for me and countless others. Your vulnerability has paved the way for many to explore new paths to health and wellness.

Barbara Williams, you have been my unwavering cheerleader through all the highs and lows. Your steadfast support and friendship have been my anchor, and I am incredibly thankful for your presence in my life. I could not ask for a better business partner or friend.

Judy Cho, your teachings about nutritional strategies, gut-healing, Chronic Inflammatory Response Syndrome (CIRS), and limbic practices have helped many people find their path to healing. Thank you for giving me the opportunity to share my story with the world.

Dr. Ritchie Shoemaker, your development of the CIRS protocol has saved countless lives, including my own. Your groundbreaking work in this field has been a beacon of hope for many, and I am profoundly grateful for your work.

To my "Meat Fam," the social media carnivore community, your support for my content and journey has been overwhelming. Your encouragement and friendship have been invaluable as I navigated this path.

Similarly, to my "CIRS Fam," the social media community of CIRS patients, your faith in my healing journey and your willingness to share in it have been a source of great motivation and strength. Your support has meant the world to me. And especially to Christian, your wisdom and courage in the face of CIRS, and your ability to give so much to others, even when you are not feeling your best, is truly inspiring.

To the team at Fair Winds Press, thank you for all your efforts in making this work a reality. Jill Alexander, thank you for guiding this book to what it is meant to be.

To Mike, thank you for believing in me and for the invaluable role you played in the creation of this book. Without your inspiration to think critically and question the status quo, it would not be what it is. And without your encouragement, it would not be.

Last but certainly not least, to Emma and Murphy, my beloved dogs. Your constant companionship and unconditional love have been a source of comfort and joy throughout this entire process. You stayed by my side through it all, including the many long hours spent writing this book.

To all of you, from the bottom of my heart, thank you. Your belief in me, your support, and your love have made this journey possible.

# NOTES

## Chapter 1: Why Carnivore?

1. Lennerz, B. S., Mey, J. T., Henn, O. H., & Ludwig, D. S. (2021). Behavioral characteristics and self-reported health status among 2029 adults consuming a "carnivore diet." *Current Developments in Nutrition*, 5(12), nzab133. https://doi.org/10.1093/cdn/nzab133.

2. Chungchunlam, S. M. S., & Moughan, P. J. (2023). Comparative bioavailability of vitamins in human foods sourced from animals and plants. *Critical Reviews in Food Science and Nutrition*, 1–36. https://doi.org/10.1080/10408398.2023.2241541.

3. Beal, T., & Ortenzi, F. (2022). Priority micronutrient density in foods. *Frontiers in Nutrition*, 9, 806566. https://doi.org/10.3389/fnut.2022.806566.

4. Home. The Weston A. Price Foundation. (n.d.). https://www.westonaprice.org/

5. Grasso, C. (2017, November 29). The Sioux. OER Commons. https://oercommons.org/authoring/25991-the-sioux.

6. Berezovikova. I. P., & Mamleeva, F. R. (2001). Traditional foods in the diet of Chukotka natives. *International Journal of Circumpolar Health*, 60:2, 138-142, DOI: 10.1080/25761900.2022.12220583.

7. Steffansson, V. (2017). *Not by Bread Alone*. Brattleboro, VT: Echo Point Books & Media. *Not by Bread Alone* by Vilhjalmur Steffansson.

8. Lennerz, B. S., Mey, J. T., Henn, O. H., & Ludwig, D. S. (2021). Behavioral Characteristics and Self-Reported Health Status among 2029 Adults Consuming a "Carnivore Diet". Current developments in nutrition, 5(12), nzab133. https://doi.org/10.1093/cdn/nzab133

9. The Weston A. Price Foundation. (n.d.). https://www.westonaprice.org.

10. Hong, Y. C. (2019). *The Changing Era of Diseases.* Cambridge, MA: Academic Press, 35–68. https://doi.org/10.1016/B978- 0-12-816439-6.00002-8.

11. Burini, R. C., & Leonard, W. R. (2018). The evolutionary roles of nutrition selection and dietary quality in the human brain size and encephalization. *Nutrire*, 43, 19. https://doi.org/10.1186/s41110-018-0078-x.

12. Lopez, M. J., & Mohiuddin, S. S. (2023). Biochemistry, essential amino acids. Treasure Island, FL: StatPearls Publishing. https://www.ncbi.nlm.nih.gov/books/NBK557845.

13. Masino, S. A., & Rho, J. M. (2012). Mechanisms of ketogenic diet action. In Noebels, J. L., Avoli, M., Rogawski, M. A., et al., eds. *Jasper's Basic Mechanisms of the Epilepsies*. 4th ed. Bethesda, MD: National Center for Biotechnology Information. https://www.ncbi.nlm.nih.gov/books/NBK98219.

14. Wilson, J. M., Lowery, R. P., Roberts, M. D., Sharp, M. H., Joy, J. M., et al. (2020). Effects of ketogenic dieting on body composition, strength, power, and hormonal profiles in resistance training men. *Journal of Strength and Conditioning Research*, 34(12): 3463-3474.

15. Pinto, A., Bonucci, A., Maggi, E., Corsi, M., & Businaro, R. (2018). Antioxidant and anti-inflammatory activity of ketogenic diet: New perspectives for neuroprotection in Alzheimer's disease. *Antioxidants*, 7(5): 63. https://doi.org/10.3390/antiox7050063.

16. Pietrzak, D., Kasperek, K., Rękawek, P., & Piątkowska-Chmiel, I. (2022). The therapeutic role of ketogenic diet in neurological disorders. *Nutrients*, 14(9): 1952. https://doi.org/10.3390/nu14091952.

17. Skolmowska, D., & Głąbska, D. (2019). Analysis of heme and non-heme iron intake and iron dietary sources in adolescent menstruating females in a national Polish sample. *Nutrients* 11(5): 1049. https://doi.org/10.3390/nu11051049.

18. NIH Office of Dietary Supplements. (n. d.). Vitamin B12. https://ods.od.nih.gov/factsheets/VitaminB12-Consumer/#:~:text=professional%20fact%2sheet.

19. NHS. Vitamin B12 or folate deficiency anaemia. (n. d.). https://www.nhs.uk/ conditions/vitamin-b12-or-folate- deficiency-anaemia.

20. Lönnerdal, B. (2000). Dietary factors influencing zinc absorption. *The Journal of Nutrition*, 130(5S Suppl): 1378S–83S. https://doi.org/10.1093/jn/130.5.1378S.

21. NIH Office of Dietary Supplements. (n. d.). Vitamin A and carotenoids. https://ods. od.nih.gov/factsheets/VitaminA-Health- Professional/#:~:text=The%20human%20diet%20contains%20two,meats%20%5B1%2C2%5D.

22. World Health Organization. (n.d.). Natural toxins in food. https://www.who.int/ news-room/fact-sheets/detail/natural- toxins-in-food.

23. Freed, D. L. (1999). Do dietary lectins cause disease? *BMJ*, 318(7190): 1023–1024. https://doi.org/10.1136/bmj.318.7190.1023.

24. Lönnerdal, B. (2000). Dietary factors influencing zinc absorption. *The Journal of Nutrition*, 130(5S Suppl): 1378S–83S. https://doi.org/10.1093/jn/130.5.1378S.

25. Di Dalmazi, G., & Cesidio, G. (2021). Plant constituents and thyroid: A revision of the main phytochemicals that interfere with thyroid function. *Food and Chemical Toxicology*, 152: 112158. https://doi.org/10.1016/j.fct.2021.112158.

26. Paśko, P., Zagrodzki, P., Okoń, K., Prochownik, E., Krośniak, M., & Galanty, A. (2022). Broccoli sprouts and their influence on thyroid function in different in vitro and in vivo models. *Plants*, 11(20): 2750. https://doi.org/10.3390/plants11202750.

27. Noonan, S. C., & Savage, G. P. (1999). Oxalate content of foods and its effect on humans. *Asia Pacific Journal of Clinical Nutrition*, 8(1): 64–74.

28. Nanayakkara, W. S., Skidmore, P. M., O'Brien, L., Wilkinson, T. J., & Gearry, R. B. (2016). Efficacy of the low FODMAP diet for treating irritable bowel syndrome: The evidence to date. *Clinical and Experimental Gastroenterology*, 9: 131–142. https://doi.org/10.2147/CEG.S86798.

29. Uhde, M., Ajamian, M., Caio, G., De Giorgio, R., Indart, A., Green, et al. (2016). Intestinal cell damage and systemic immune activation in individuals reporting sensitivity to wheat in the absence of coeliac disease. *Gut*, 65(12): 1930–1937. https://doi.org/10.1136/gutjnl-2016-311964.

30. Kęszycka, P. K., Lange, E., & Gajewska, D. (2021). Effectiveness of personalized low salicylate diet in the management of salicylates hypersensitive patients: Interventional study. *Nutrients*, 13(3): 991. https://doi.org/10.3390/nu13030991.

31. Tudi, M., Li, H., Li, H., Wang, L., Lyu, J., Yang, L., et al. (2022). Exposure routes and health risks associated with pesticide application. *Toxics*, 10(6): 335. https://doi.org/10.3390/toxics10060335.

32. Federico, A., Rosato, V., Masarone, M., Torre, P., Dallio, M., Romeo, M., & Persico, M. (2021). The role of fructose in nonalcoholic steatohepatitis: Old relationship and new insights. *Nutrients*, 13(4): 1314. https://doi.org/10.3390/nu13041314.

33. Armstrong, H. K., Bording-Jorgensen, M., Santer, D. M., Zhang, Z., Valcheva, R., Rieger, A. M., et al. (2023). Unfermented β-fructan fibers fuel inflammation in select inflammatory bowel disease patients. *Gastroenterology*, 164(2): 228–240. https://doi.org/10.1053/j.gastro.2022.09.034.

34. Lennerz, B. S., Mey, J. T., Henn, O. H., & Ludwig, D. S. (2021). Behavioral characteristics and self-reported health status among 2029 adults consuming a "carnivore diet." *Current Developments in Nutrition*, 5(12): nzab133. https://doi.org/10.1093/cdn/nzab133.

35. Ibid.

36. Ibid.

37. Cho, K. H. (2022). The current status of research on high-density lipoproteins (HDL): A paradigm shift from HDL quantity to HDL quality and HDL functionality. *International Journal of Molecular Sciences*, 23(7): 3967. https://doi.org/10.3390/ijms23073967.

38. Cleveland Clinic. (n. d.). What is inflammation? https://my.clevelandclinic.org/health/symptoms/21660-inflammation.

39. Loh, W., & Tang, M. L. K. (2018). The epidemiology of food allergy in the global context. *International Journal of Environmental Research and Public Health*, 15(9): 2043. https://doi.org/10.3390/ijerph15092043.

40. Di Corcia, M., Tartaglia, N., Polito, R., Ambrosi, A., Messina, G., et al. (2022). Functional properties of meat in athletes' performance and recovery. *International Journal of Environmental Research and Public Health*, 19(9): 5145. https://doi.org/10.3390/ijerph19095145.

41. Ouabbou, S., He, Y., Butler, K., & Tsuang, M. (2020). Inflammation in mental disorders: Is the microbiota the missing link? *Neuroscience Bulletin*, 36(9): 1071–1084. https://doi.org/10.1007/s12264-020-00535-1.

42. Bandelow, B., & Michaelis, S. (2015). Epidemiology of anxiety disorders in the 21st century. *Dialogues in Clinical Neuroscience*, 17(3): 327–335. https://doi.org/10.31887/DCNS.2015.17.3/bbandelow.

43. Norwitz, N. G., & Naidoo, U. (2021). Nutrition as metabolic treatment for anxiety. *Frontiers in Psychiatry*, 12: 598119. https://doi.org/10.3389/fpsyt.2021.598119.

44. Won, E., & Kim, Y. K. (2020). Neuroinflammation-associated alterations of the brain as potential neural biomarkers in anxiety disorders. *International Journal of Molecular Sciences*, 21(18): 6546. https://doi.org/10.3390/ijms21186546.

45. Yang, T., Velagapudi, R., Kong, C., Ko, U., Kumar, V., et al. (2023). Protective effects of omega-3 fatty acids in a blood-brain barrier-on-chip model and on postoperative delirium-like behaviour in mice. *British Journal of Anaesthesia*, 130(2): e370–e380. https://doi.org/10.1016/j.bja.2022.05.025.

46. Basiri, R., Seidu, B., & Rudich, M. (2023). Exploring the interrelationships between diabetes, nutrition, anxiety, and depression: Implications for treatment and prevention strategies. *Nutrients*, 15(19): 4226. https://doi.org/10.3390/nu15194226.

47. Fiani, B., Zhu, L., Musch, B. L., Briceno, S., Andel, R., et al. (2021). The neurophysiology of caffeine as a central nervous system stimulant and the resultant effects on cognitive function. *Cureus*, 13(5): e15032. https://doi.org/10.7759/cureus.15032.

48. Valentine, G., & Sofuoglu, M. (2018). Cognitive effects of nicotine: Recent progress. *Current Neuropharmacology*, 16(4): 403–414. https://doi.org/10.2174/1570159X15666171103152136.

49. Zahra, S., Hossein, S., & Ali, K. V. (2012). Relationship between opium abuse and severity of depression in type 2 diabetic patients. *Diabetes & Metabolism Journal*, 36(2): 157-162. https://doi.org/10.4093/dmj.2012.36.2.157.

50. Gordon, E. L., Ariel-Donges, A. H., Bauman, V., & Merlo, L. J. (2018). What is the evidence for "food addiction?" A systematic review. *Nutrients*, 10(4): 477. https://doi.org/10.3390/nu10040477.

51. Vasiliu, O. (2022). Current status of evidence for a new diagnosis: Food addiction—a literature review. *Frontiers in Psychiatry*, 12: 824936. https://doi.org/10.3389/fpsyt.2021.824936.

52. Rubin, G. (2022). Back by popular demand: Are you an abstainer or a moderator? https://gretchenrubin.com/articles/abstainer-vs-moderator.

## Chapter 2: What Is Carnivore?

53. Song, D. K., & Kim, Y. W. (2023). Beneficial effects of intermittent fasting: A narrative review. *Journal of Yeungnam Medical Science*, 40(1): 4–11. https://doi.org/10.12701/jyms.2022.00010.

54. D'Andrea Meira, I., Romão, T. T., Pires do Prado, H. J., Krüger, L. T., Pires, M. E. P., & da Conceição, P. O. (2019). Ketogenic diet and epilepsy: What we know so far. *Frontiers in Neuroscience*, 13, 5. https://doi.org/10.3389/fnins.2019.00005

55. Solan, M. (2023, December 18). How healthy is sugar alcohol? Harvard Health. https://www.health.harvard.edu/blog/how-healthy-is-sugar-alcohol-202312183002#:~:text=The%20downside%20of%20sugar%20alcohols&text=Because%20sugar%20alcohols%20are%20slowly,and%20cause%20a%20laxative%20effect.

56. Spooner, H. C., Derrick, S. A., Maj, M., Manjarín, R., Hernandez, G. V., et al. (2021). High-fructose, high-fat diet alters muscle composition and fuel utilization in a juvenile Iberian pig model of non-alcoholic fatty liver disease. *Nutrients*, 13(12): 4195. https://doi.org/10.3390/nu13124195.

57. Poznyak, A. V., Litvinova, L., Poggio, P., Sukhorukov, V. N., & Orekhov, A. N. (2022). Effect of glucose levels on cardiovascular risk. *Cells*, 11(19): 3034. https://doi.org/10.3390/cells11193034.

58. Olson, J. M., Ameer, M. A., & Goyal, A. (2024). Vitamin A Toxicity. Treasure Island, FL: StatPearls Publishing. https://www.ncbi.nlm.nih.gov/books/NBK532916.

59. Astrup, A., Teicholz, N., Magkos, F., Bier, D. M., Brenna, J. T., et al. (2021). Dietary saturated fats and health: Are the U.S. guidelines evidence-based? *Nutrients*, 13(10): 3305. https://doi.org/10.3390/nu13103305.

60. Ibid.

61. Soliman, G. A. (2018). Dietary cholesterol and the lack of evidence in cardiovascular disease. *Nutrients*, 10(6): 780. https://doi.org/10.3390/nu10060780.

62. NIH Office of Dietary Supplements. (n. d.). Vitamin and mineral supplement fact sheets. https://ods.od.nih.gov/factsheets/list-VitaminsMinerals.

63. Mack, J. (2019, November 15). Police say footage PETA claimed was from Indiana pig farm may have been staged. *The Indianapolis Star*. https://www.indystar.com/story/news/crime/2019/11/14/peta-footage-indiana-farm-may-have-been-faked- police-say/4192340002.

64. Fischer, Bob & Lamey, Andy (2018). Field Deaths in Plant Agriculture. *Journal of Agricultural and Environmental Ethics* 31 (4):409-428.

65. Beal, T., & Ortenzi, F. (2022). Priority micronutrient density in foods. *Frontiers in Nutrition*, 9, 806566. https://doi.org/10.3389/fnut.2022.806566.

66. Fischer, B., & Lamey, A. (2018). Field deaths in plant agriculture. *Journal of Agricultural and Environmental Ethics*, 31: 409–428. https://doi.org/10.1007/s10806-018-9733-8.

## Chapter 3: How to Transition to a Carnivore Diet

67. Strasser, B., Volaklis, K., Fuchs, D., & Burtscher, M. (2018). Role of dietary protein and muscular fitness on longevity and aging. *Aging and Disease*, 9(1): 119–132. https://doi.org/10.14336/AD.2017.0202.

68. Center for Food Safety and Applied Nutrition. (n. d.). How to understand and use the nutrition facts label. https://www.fda.gov/food/nutrition-facts-label/how-understand-and-use-nutrition-facts-label.

69. Shabkhizan, R., Haiaty, S., Moslehian, M. S., Bazmani, A., Sadeghsoltani, F., et al. (2023). The beneficial and adverse effects of autophagic response to caloric restriction and fasting. *Advances in Nutrition*, 14(5): 1211–1225. https://doi.org/10.1016/j.advnut.2023.07.006.

70. Aly, S. M. (2014). Role of intermittent fasting on improving health and reducing diseases. *International Journal of Health Sciences*, 8(3): V–VI. https://doi.org/10.12816/0023985.

71. Palmblad, J., Hafström, I., & Ringertz, B. (1991). Antirheumatic effects of fasting. *Rheumatic Diseases Clinics of North America*, 17(2): 351–362.

72. Gröber, U., Werner, T., Vormann, J., & Kisters, K. (2017). Myth or reality—transdermal magnesium? *Nutrients*, 9(8): 813. https://doi.org/10.3390/nu9080813.

73. Singh, M., & Mukhopadhyay, K. (2014). Alpha-melanocyte stimulating hormone: An emerging anti-inflammatory antimicrobial peptide. *BioMed Research International*, 874610. https://doi.org/10.1155/2014/874610.

74. Sizar, O., Khare, S., Goyal, A., et al. (2024). Vitamin D deficiency. Treasure Island, FL: StatPearls Publishing. https://www.ncbi.nlm.nih.gov/books/NBK532266.

75. Raymond-Lezman, J. R., & Riskin, S. I. (2023). Benefits and risks of sun exposure to maintain adequate vitamin D levels. *Cureus*, 15(5): e38578. https://doi.org/10.7759/cureus.38578.

76. Cho, C. H., Yoon, H. K., Kang, S. G., Kim, L., Lee, E. I., & Lee, H. J. (2018). Impact of exposure to dim light at night on sleep in female and comparison with male subjects. *Psychiatry Investigation*, 15(5): 520–530. https://doi.org/10.30773/pi.2018.03.17.

## Chapter 4: Overcoming Obstacles to Your Success on a Carnivore Diet

77. Scott, R. F. (1905). *The Voyage of the Discovery*. London: Cooper Sqaure Press, 541–545 [September 26, 1902] [The expedition members] Heald, Mr. Ferrar, and Cross have very badly swollen legs, whilst Heald's are discoloured as well. The remainder of the party seem fairly well, but not above suspicion; Walker's ankles are slightly swollen. [October 15, 1902] [After a fresh seal meat diet at base camp] within a fortnight of the outbreak there is scarcely a sign of it remaining . . . Heald's is the only case that hung at all . . . and now he is able to get about once more. Cross's recovery was so rapid that he was able to join the seal-killing party last week.

78. Sweis, I. E., & Cressey, B. C. (2018). Potential role of the common food additive manufactured citric acid in eliciting significant inflammatory reactions contributing to serious disease states: A series of four case reports. *Toxicology Reports*, 5: 808–812. https://doi.org/10.1016/j.toxrep.2018.08.002.

79. Montgomery, D. R., Biklé, A., Archuleta, R., Brown, P., & Jordan, J. (2022). Soil health and nutrient density: Preliminary comparison of regenerative and conventional farming. *PeerJ*, 10: e12848. https://doi.org/10.7717/peerj.12848.

80. Chao, H. W., Chao, S. W., Lin, H., Ku, H. C., & Cheng, C. F. (2019). Homeostasis of Glucose and Lipid in Non-Alcoholic Fatty Liver Disease. *International journal of molecular sciences*, 20(2), 298. https://doi.org/10.3390/ijms20020298

81. National Institute on Aging. (n. d.). Research on intermittent fasting shows health benefits. https://www.nia.nih.gov/news/research-intermittent-fasting-shows-health-benefits#:~:text=Hundreds%20of%20animal%20studies%20and,less%20clear%20for%20lifespan%20effects.

82. https://criticalcarnivore.netlify.app/4.

83. Clapp, M., Aurora, N., Herrera, L., Bhatia, M., Wilen, E., & Wakefield, S. (2017). Gut microbiota's effect on mental health: The gut-brain axis. *Clinics and Practice*, 7(4): 987. https://doi.org/10.4081/cp.2017.987.

84. Eisenhofer, G., Åneman, A., Friberg, P., Hooper, D., Fåndriks, L., et al. (1997). Substantial production of dopamine in the human gastrointestinal tract. *The Journal of Clinical Endocrinology & Metabolism*, 82(11): 3864–3871. https://doi.org/10.1210/jcem.82.11.4339.

85. Campbell, A. W. (2014). Autoimmunity and the gut. *Autoimmune Diseases*, 2014, 152428. https://doi.org/10.1155/2014/152428.

86. Lennerz, B. S., Mey, J. T., Henn, O. H., & Ludwig, D. S. (2021). Behavioral characteristics and self-reported health status among 2029 adults consuming a "carnivore diet." *Current Developments in Nutrition*, 5(12): nzab133. https://doi.org/10.1093/cdn/nzab133.

87. Wang, Y., Uffelman, C. N., Bergia, R. E., Clark, C. M., Reed, J. B., et. al. (2023). Meat consumption and gut microbiota: A scoping review of literature and systematic review of randomized controlled trials in adults. *Advances in Nutrition*, 14(2): 215–237. https://doi.org/10.1016/j.advnut.2022.10.005.

88. Ekirch, A. R. (2016). Segmented sleep in preindustrial societies. *Sleep*, 39(3): 715–716. https://pubmed.ncbi.nlm.nih.gov/26888454.

89. Lennerz, B. S., Mey, J. T., Henn, O. H., & Ludwig, D. S. (2021). Behavioral characteristics and self-reported health status among 2029 adults consuming a "carnivore diet." *Current Developments in Nutrition*, 5(12): nzab133. https://doi.org/10.1093/cdn/nzab133.

## Chapter 5: Off-Boarding from a Carnivore Diet

90. Fedewa, A., & Rao, S. S. (2014). Dietary fructose intolerance, fructan intolerance and FODMAPs. *Current Gastroenterology Reports*, 16(1): 370. https://doi.org/10.1007/s11894-013-0370-0.

91. National Institutes of Health. (2020). How high fructose intake may trigger fatty liver disease. https://www.nih.gov/news-events/nih-research-matters/how-high-fructose-intake-may-trigger-fatty-liver-disease.

# INDEX